# Endorsements

*Life Is a Circus; Enjoy the Show* is a story of a real woman sharing how she left behind a dimly lit, ordinary life for a life of courage, fun, magic, and real success.

Angela Witczak's inner flame burns so brightly that all who surround her are caught up in the blaze. There is nothing more courageous than surviving and thriving on the other side of struggle. This book exemplifies how overcoming heartbreak and obstacles are the keys to a full life.

—The Fabulous Dorris Burch
Transformation coach at Fab Factor, best-selling
author of *The Little Black Book of Being Fabulous* and
*Don't Be Invisible Be Fabulous* anthology book series.
Hostess of the New Fab Your Show Podcast

Angela Witczak gives us ring side seats to her real life in an authentic and vulnerable way. Many authors will tip-toe through raw stuff in their lives. Angela not only takes it head-on, but she holds up a mirror for the readers to see themselves in her story. If you are still twisted up in self-judgement over choices, you have made in your life this book is a must read.

—Laura Hulleman
Creator of the Endotype Formula
www.endotype.com

# LIFE IS A CIRCUS

Enjoy the Show

ANGELA WITCZAK

Printed in the United States of America

Published by Author Academy Elite
P.O. Box 43, Powell, OH 43035

326 Badger Drive Baraboo WI 53913.
choosetoday366@gmail.com.
www.choosetoday366.com

Paperback: 978-1-64746-731-9
Hardback: 978-1-64746-732-6
E-book: 978-1-64746-733-3
(LCCN): 2021903668

# Dedication

For my husband:
Thank you for never giving up on me. From day one when
you chose to follow me around a grocery store, until now
2,853 days later—when you continue to follow me around
our house. You have pursued my heart with a never-ending
tenacity and strength. From our worst days to our best days,
you have never left my side. I will always be your beautiful
mess that you chose.
I love you Ward.

For all of my children:
You are *my* Circus! You bring me great joy every single day.

And for Laura,
You told me two years ago,
*"Just write the damn book!"*
And I did.
Enjoy.

# Foreward

*Life Is a Circus: Enjoy the Show* is a must-read for anyone who desires to become the Ringmaster of their life!

Who doesn't love the circus: the excitement, entertainment, edge-of-your-seat action that takes place along with the exotic animals and fun-filled atmosphere under the Big Top? Most people enjoy watching death-defying acrobatics, lion tamers, and especially laughing at those silly clowns. It brings joy.

However, this isn't true when your life *becomes the circus* and life's lions get out of control, or you become the sad clown.

If anyone understands the phrase, "Life is a circus," it's Angela. Her life has resembled a three-ring circus on more than one occasion. However, she has found a way to enjoy the show amidst the chaos, confusion, and even life calamities. She has taken these truths and strategies that have helped her overcome the struggles many of you face and show you how to overcome life's obstacles.

You will see behind the curtain as she reveals the truth about her experiences, allowing you the amazing opportunity to glean from her times of calamity as well as her times of courage. Using analogies from the circus and applying them to life, you will find her relevant and transformational teachings.

If you struggle with juggling the chaos, taming those ferocious lions, feeling like a clown, or simply trying to be the strong person in your life, Angela understands and will help you find peace, joy, and forgiveness in the chaos of life. This book will allow you to move through the ranks until you find yourself as the Ringmaster of your circus.

Time has also been compared to the circus, always packing up and moving away, so I encourage you to take the time to read this book, not allowing anything or anyone else to be the Ringmaster of your life any longer.

—Jody Almond
CEO of Soulution Ministries/author of Going
All In-Finding Success Through Surrender / Life
and Business Coach/ Motivational Speaker

# Table of Contents

# Introduction

When most folks state their *life is a circus*, they are actually saying there is chaos ensuing throughout every corner. Your circus might look a little like this:

You are tired and sleep-deprived from your baby, who has gotten up numerous times through the night to eat. Your toddler has asked you for the nine-millionth time if he can have a snack, meanwhile spilling all of the cheerios he currently has—on the ground, again. Your teenager is in a love/hate relationship with you. She only loves you when you are giving her money or rides and pretty much hates you all of the rest of the time. You are tired, and your husband keeps looking at you from across the room, with *the look,* and you are avoiding eye contact because all you want is to shower and wash your hair by yourself—with no interruptions from anyone. The dog peed on the floor again, for the third time this week, and someone has to clean it up—more than likely that someone is you.

Is that the circus you remember as a child growing up, or was it a little different?

• • •

When I was a little girl, about five years old, my parents took me to the circus. My grandparents lived in Baraboo, Wisconsin which is the home to the *Ringling Brothers and Barnum Bailey Circus*. I would play in their backyard with the music of the calliope to guide my play. There is something so magical about being little and hearing circus music.

One beautiful summer day, my mother told me that she was going to take me to the circus. She put me into an adorable red and white polka-dotted dress and put little pig tails in my hair. Outside the circus' gates were garbage cans that looked like clowns, with grinning faces, welcoming us in.

The circus in Baraboo, Wisconsin, is different than traveling circuses—the Big Top was set up all summer long. You could see the large red and white stripes of the tent from the road, beckoning us to come and see the show. My tiny 5-year-old self was bursting with anticipation of what I would see there.

When you are five, everything seems so big, magical, and enticing. The circus smelled of cotton candy, popcorn, and manure from the animals. Everywhere I looked there were vibrant colors, sounds, and things to see. Loud, jovial music was playing in the background throughout the grounds. Large, beautiful circus posters and train wagons adorned with pictures of different oddities and performers for the upcoming shows were everywhere.

Not only was this a circus complete with performances, but it was also a museum—the Circus World Museum.[1] There was a miniature circus exhibit that would be my favorite piece of the museum in the years to come. I would push all of the display's little buttons to make each part move and show off different aspects of the circus. Like magic, the tiny horses would move to the water trough, or the small toy men would construct the Big Top with mallets, and the lion tamer would move his tiny whip up and down. It was a wonderous display, which still stands today (only without the moving parts and buttons).

My mother was an expert at navigating the circus schedule to see all of the different programs. My favorite program, besides the Big Top, was the clown show. A man would put on clown makeup and transform right in front of my very eyes. He would go from a sweet older man to the funniest clown, and no matter how many times I saw that program throughout the years, I was continually transformed right along with him into a new character.

We would make our trek over to the Big Top from the clown show, where a fantastic menagerie waited for us in the entryway. I was able to see exotic animals, up close, for the very first time in my life: a giraffe as tall as the tent, an ostrich full of feathers, goats, snakes, performing dogs, and even a black panther in a cage! We would stand in line waiting to look at all of these exotics while impatiently hoping they would lower the rope-gate for us to enter.

In my early years of going to the circus, just being at the circus was enough. There was no need for all of the extras, like circus treats or souvenirs, because I knew in my own way that we didn't have a lot of money. My mother would bring along a tiny cooler, and before the show would start, she would hand each of my brothers and me a small barrel-shaped juice and other treats she had brought along with her. The food vendors would be walking around hollering, "Cotton candy, get your cotton candy here! Popcorn! Hot buttered popcorn!" I knew enough not to ask for those extra treats, however, the vendors were amusing to watch.

I would sit on the hard bleachers inside the sweaty tent and watch all the people filter in through the entrance. People who dressed extra fancy always sat ringside. They had the best view in the whole place. I often wished I was as famous as those people. I found out much later in life, those seats cost money, and usually, it was just people who could afford to sit there, no fame or recognition required.

I talked and pointed out everything and everybody as they came in! "Look at that over there! Wow—look at the band! I wonder what songs they will play! He has the drums! Look, there is a trumpet! Mom! Look—there and there and there!"

My mother would "shush" me, and then I would wait for the show to start. The man I saw who transformed into the same funny clown would come out and do some silly, entertaining tricks. He had a little dog with him, and it was so amusing to see him jumping up and down, rolling over, and then playing dead!

And then, I would hear it. The whistle. The whistle that told the audience to take their seats—one minute until show time! The whistle was like a secret code signaling the significant start of the show. The vendors would make their way down the bleachers and back over to the food carts, and we would all wait. And then, the second whistle. That whistle announced the start of the show!

There was a huge band on the band stand, and it would start to play with the ringing of the trumpets, the drums, and the clashing of the symbols hitting the audience with exciting energy. With bated breath, I would wait. Finally, the Ringmaster would come in with his microphone and sing the most amazing songs welcoming us to the show. The performers with giant head pieces, animals on parade, jugglers, and all of the acts would come in through the tent curtains for a huge opening number. My very first glimpse at a LIVE show. My first taste at seeing what was to happen over the next ninety minutes.

Even though I was just five years old, I would sit quietly and watch each act with great enthusiasm and interest. The way the juggler would throw bowling balls into the air and catch them, never dropping them or even buckling under the weight. He would carefully and yet very daringly toss batons made of fire, being cautious not to scorch himself and then add more bowling pins than my little eyes could count. It was so magical to me the way he flipped and tossed juggling rings into the air. The greatest trick of all, he would flip them all over, revealing color on one side—white on the other, and then black! How did he even do that?

As quickly as the juggler would come out, he would be done with his act and on to the next one. I gasped along with the rest of the crowd as the tightrope act performed high above my head. I closed my eyes and hoped for the best as they rode forward and backward on a bicycle. And when the rest of the crowd clapped, I knew I could look again and that the performer was okay!

However, then, he would start jumping rope and would beckon us to cheer him on! He would pump his arm up and down to signal to the audience to cheer louder and louder—each trick more and more daring than the last. Finally, he would hold up a blindfold—a blindfold! With his eyes covered, he attempted to jump the rope with no ability to see. My stomach would drop to my knees and I would cover my eyes as well (but I would peek out through my fingers to see if he made it).

He did it! The crowd would cheer and scream in joy for him as he walked to the side platform and then would attempt a slide for his life down the side wire! Every trick that he did seemed more exciting than the last, and my heart felt like it would burst from pure excitement.

Suddenly, there was that crazy clown again. He rushed out into the arena walking around roasting a hot dog. The Ringmaster would come running out after him yelling, "There's no smoking in the ring!" And he would chase him out. The music would speed up and slow down while the chase was happening to make all of us laugh.

Acrobats and other stunts were next to enter the ring. But my favorite act, even as a little girl, was the elephants.

The Ringmaster would announce them by saying, "Hold your horses, here come the elephants!"

These ginormous creatures did stunts that astounded me. The giant pachyderms seemed graceful as they came in by parade, tail to trunk. They would get midway into the ring and perform a spin as they would walk around. They would climb up onto bull stands and spin around with their hind legs on the frame and their front legs on the ground. The music would move right along with them! Finally, the trick that everyone waited for—the Elephant Long mount! The first elephant stayed on the ground, while the other elephants lifted their front legs up onto the next elephant's back, and they lifted their trunks high in the air. It is truly magnificent!

The elephants would leave the ring, and we would all clap and cheer. The show was winding down. The only thing left would be the final curtain call for the performers and some of the animals. They would parade through the back curtain, singing and waving flags. The Ringmaster would sing the final number. As the last note rang out, he would thank us for coming and say, "May all your days be circus days!"

We would file out of the Big Top feeling happy and over-whelmed with joy—ready to see the *Side Show*. There was a small tent set up of statues from PT Barnum's *Side Show* from years gone by. There were statues of famous people who were known for being *Circus Freaks*: A man covered in hair, a set of Siamese twins connected in their sternum, a small man who we all knew as Tom Thumb, and a statue of the fat lady. We would walk through the tent, and my mother would point out the different oddities and read the informa-tion about each one.

We would walk past the elephants that were giving rides and head over to a grassy spot next to the train of historic circus wagons and a merry-go-round. It was near the river, and it was such a beautiful place where we could see all of the different things happening around us.

My mother always brought the same lunch during the years we visited the circus: ham sandwiches, pringles, and juice boxes. It was a special picnic lunch that we only had when we went on these little field trips. In my memories, it was one of the best lunches I ever had.

After we would finish eating, my brothers and I would spin each other on the merry-go-round. Round and round, we would go until one of us felt sick. After lunch, we'd walk around the wagon building and look at all of the different historic circus wagons. A couple of wagon cars were open for us to walk through and see what it was like to live on a circus train.

After lunch, there was one final show—the illusion show. It was featured in the Hippodrome building that was always set up year-round (unlike the circus tent). Entering the building, I saw sawdust covering the ground, a stage, bleachers, and the small ring where children could sit.

The magic tricks always blew away my tiny mind. My favorite trick was called the *Dancing Handkerchief*. The magician would ask an audience member for a clean white handkerchief to be used in the act, and then he would make it do the most amazing tricks. The hanky would move along to the music from the Pink Panther. The handkerchief would fly across the stage through hoops, lay down, and jump up in the air at the hand of the magician, all in time with the music. To this day, I will never know how that trick is done, nor do I want to know.

As the final illusion came to an end, so did our magical circus trip. My heart would be bursting with joy at the day that we had and feel sad simultaneously as we left the beloved circus. With heavy feet, we crossed the bridge and headed to the parking lot. Sitting in the car waiting for the crowds to go, I felt my happiness slide into a frown, and yet, I knew there was a spark of hope. The following year, we would return to do it all again.

This is the memory of my childhood. The memory that reminds me as to why the circus is called the *Greatest Place on Earth*. It evokes magic, joy, and bittersweet memories of all the world's good and positive things.

It's what I imagine life to be like when I hear people say their *life is a circus*. However, I am guessing if you picked up this book thinking not of all the positive things in your life but the chaotic things, you are in the right place.

I am here to tell you that you are not alone. I invite you to come along with me as I show you how I lived in this proverbial circus. How I experienced never-ending grief, sadness, and sorrow, and how through each bit of the trials, I was able to find joy sprinkled throughout my life—like the magic that happens at the circus. Come along with me as we journey through the challenging topics of death, disease, divorce, and even adoption, and at the end of the day, I still call my life the *Greatest Show on Earth*.

# ••• CHAPTER 1 •••
# The Fat Lady

IN THE EARLY 1900's when touring circuses were the biggest form of entertainment, it was well known that along with the acts came side show oddities. There were the sword swallowers, the dwarf-sized men, the Siamese twins, and of course, the Fat lady.

The interesting part about *fat ladies* (in the circus) was that they were the only side show freak who could actually control what people found weird about them—their weight. Unlike someone who carried a gene that made them incredibly short or covered in hair, people who are overweight can, in fact, lose weight.

In the 1930's one of the most well-known circus fat women, Celesta Geyer, was the famous Dolly Dimples. She topped the scales at almost 588 pounds and was known not only for her weight but incredible singing voice. She started gaining weight when she was just a girl because of her love for food and abuse she suffered from her family. By the time she was in her mid-twenties, she had weighed almost 400 pounds. She then traveled with the circus until she was almost 40 years old—until her weight became too much for her to allow her to travel. Years later, she had a near-fatal heart attack.[1]

• • •

I understand, my dear friend Dolly Dimples, because I have always been the *fat girl*. Can you relate to that? Maybe you weren't the *fat girl* though, perhaps you were the one that they always called scrawny or weak, or you were the *pretty one with no brains*. Bottom line, you always felt a little out of place—like someone who belonged in a side show. For me, I was the *fat girl*.

I wasn't always overweight. In the second grade, my pictures show that I was a cute little petite girl. Maybe I weighed 45 pounds. I have no idea. All I know is that when I was in the second grade, as a little girl, I was cute, adorable and small. And then somewhere between my second-grade school picture and my third-grade picture, I became the fat kid.

I was the *fat girl.*

It is easy to look back now on my life and understand why I was packing on all of those pounds. My family was in the military and right around that time in my life was the first real move that I could actually remember. I don't have any recollections of the stories that my parents told me of the times that we lived in Germany, where I was born, or in Kentucky, where my brother was born. I only know that Leland, Wisconsin, was my first real home.

My parents came home from work when I was about seven and informed me that we were moving. My mother had gotten a teaching job six hours north. She was going to be a computer teacher—whatever that was—I had no idea. I grew up in the 80s, and we didn't have computers, smart phones, iPads or any other technology. I grew up in the era where you played outside until the streetlights came on.

Two weeks into my third-grade year, my parents packed up all of our belongings, and we moved to the northernmost part of Wisconsin. I started in a new school where I stuck out like a sore thumb.

For anyone that knows me personally, they know that I pretty much don't ever keep my mouth shut, and even back then I was no different. At the new school, I was always getting in trouble for talking. Even when the teacher had her back to the class, if someone was talking, I was generally to blame for it. I stuck out like a sideshow freak.

Being the new kid in my hand-me-down clothes, I didn't really have many friends, so like most kids, I ate my feelings—hence, the *fat girl*.

For most of my childhood, I was the butt of other kids' jokes. When we would move to a new town, I felt like the poor kid, with my thrift store clothing and being much too large for my own good. There I was, always standing out—too loud, too obnoxious, and too fat.

There have only been two times in my whole life that I can remember being *thin*, aside from the second grade, of course. Twice more we moved, and the second time was in the midst of my 8th grade year of middle school. While I was the fat girl, I was also the smart kid. I had buried myself in books throughout much of my early junior high years, and I was incredibly intelligent. So, when we moved to this new school, I was put in *advanced classes*.

All that meant was now I was the underdog, with kids that were older than me. The added insult was that they were even ruder than what I was used to. I showed them all, though, by doing what any smart kid would do and got the highest grade on the class tests. I would act like their jokes about how enormous my back side was didn't bother me, but wow, did it hurt!

After that school year was over, I was heading to the high school level, 9th grade. That is when I lost some weight. I hit puberty and grew several inches. I was too young to drive, so, I walked everywhere I wanted to hang out with friends. I went from the hefty size 18 that I had been, to a size 10. That might not seem very small to some of you, but for me, that was truly thin.

I often felt like I was too big and bulky for my skin. I stayed that desired size for a while. And then, like all teenagers do, I went through my first major heartbreak, with the first love of my life, and the weight came back on. Like any teenage girl, I drowned my sorrows in the like of pints of Ben and Jerry's ice cream and Beverly Hills 90210. Jason Priestley satisfied my heart desires, so there was no need to be thin any longer.

I stayed very overweight for many years. Almost a protection that I was keeping for myself. People couldn't hurt me if they couldn't get close enough to me to break my heart. Obviously, though, I did let people into my heart and life. I fell in love with a man that was also overweight. He was considered grossly obese at that time, as much as the great Dolly Dimples even.

As I couldn't see past my own size and thinking that I was never worthy of having someone love me that was not overweight, I married this man. My weight was a constant and consistent struggle throughout our entire marriage.

I had people that had made comments to me. That maybe I would be happier if I lost some weight. My *was-band* (that's the name I came up with for my previous husband), and I even tried a few times to lose weight; we were just unsuccessful. With all the pressure I constantly felt, I carried around a lot of internal baggage about my weight.

I felt like my weight kept me from having friendships with people who were prettier and thinner than myself. Internally, I felt as though I was being judged at all times. I would go to places with people I knew, and every time I would brace myself for the negative judgment I carried around. I never went shopping when my friends asked me. Why would I? I would have to try on something that didn't fit and then carry that embarrassment and shame around. I did not want other people to see my struggle or my weight. It felt like my worst nightmare.

It wasn't until my marriage was on the brink of ruins that I decided maybe if I was just prettier (by being skinnier), my husband would love me. If I just weighed a few pounds less, then he, and everyone else, would think higher of me. I would be one of those *pretty skinny girls*.

I wanted to be liked by others. I wanted to be able to look into the mirror and like what I saw. That was the biggest thing that was killing me every day. I wanted to be beautiful, which meant *I wanted to be thin*.

Most of all, though, I wanted my *was-band* to really love me. I wanted him to desire me. I thought that by losing weight, I could magically fix our marriage and fix him— then I could finally have a great relationship. Even though he was still overweight, I knew if I lost the weight, I could be thin enough for both of us, and our problems would go away. Suddenly we would be happier. I totally ignored the fact that we had issues much more significant than my weight or his weight. Our problems were deep, and they cut through the heart.

One day, I made the decision. I was going to lose weight, no matter what. I found a personal trainer and a small gym that I loved. And I started losing weight. Every morning, I would get up, and I would rush to the bathroom. I would take my clothes off, and I would step on the scale. I would hold my breath as I waited to see what those numbers would have for me.

Was I going to have a good day or a bad day? Well, that all depended on what the scale said. Every morning, I lived and breathed by whatever the scale said. If the number was not as good, I would work out a little harder that day, if the number was better, then maybe I could forgive that little *cheat* of a cookie. I ended up losing over sixty pounds that year.

My body transformed over six months. I worked hard at losing weight. I was learning how to eat healthy and how to be in shape. Near the end of the six months, I became a Zumba instructor and started working out about twenty hours every single week. I lived in the gym. Now, I know you are all dying to know. Did it work? Did my *was-band* stick around and our marriage improve? Well, here are your answers:

- Did the weight coming off fix my marriage? No.
- Did the weight coming off make me fall in love with myself? No.
- Did I continue to hear negative things from other people? Yes.

That is the thing—the negativity didn't stop! I didn't actually change anything at all, except for my outsides. The size of my jeans was terrific, however, I still ached internally.

I went from being the *fat girl* to now the negative things that were being said about me were,

"I was losing too much weight."

"I only got hot, so I could leave my husband."

"I look ridiculous wearing workout clothes every day."

"I was just *too much* for my friends."

There were a lot of things that I heard over the days and weeks as I was on my journey to weight loss and self-discovery. And do you know what? The very same people that had encouraged me to lose weight, were now the ones destroying my newfound skinniness. (See how you can't please anyone).

Comments like those propelled me back to my childhood and the pain that went with it. I would always be the *whale of a girl* or that *maybe I should get a second helping because I was so fat, and I needed more to eat.*

● ● ●

Childhood: this is where we start forming our ideas of who we are. We begin to tell ourselves *they said it; it must be true—* this is who I am. As we get older and we continue to hear those nasty remarks in our heads. They seem to validate what we already believe about ourselves.

"And now, welcome to the chaos of a piece of circus in your head. For my next act, I bring to all of you, *The Scale!*" I allowed it to continually validate my weight and my over-weight-ness for me.

But the thing is, my dear friends, that was a lie I was telling myself.

Let me say this again, maybe for the people in the back row to truly hear this, what other people say or believe about us, is often a *LIE*. Everyone else on this planet will tell you something that you either WANT to hear about yourself, or something that *they* want to hear about *themselves*. They are going to tear you down for the very same reasons. People often bring to light the very thing that they themselves are struggling with. It is so easy to recognize the same character flaw in another person, if we are challenged with the same thing, right?

Think of it like those distorted mirrors you see sometimes at the circus. You look at them, and you see your head is too big for your body, or vice versa. What other people say about you, is often just like that. They are reflecting back to you what they see in themselves, not in you. Which is why so often, it's their truth they are speaking, not yours.

It's easy to sit around with a group of women and discuss all of the things that are wrong with your husbands or kids, because many of us share the same struggles. They don't pick up their toys, or our husbands like to watch too much football on Sundays while we are picking up after everyone and planning our week, or the dog peed on the floor again. It's easy to identify with others or recognize faults in others the very same way.

Personally, I struggle with self-esteem. That's what the crux of this chapter is about. It is far easier for me to recognize when another woman is struggling with her weight or appearance than it is for me to identify other traits, such as leadership, because I find that is something I am fairly good at.

When I changed my own thinking about who I was, the weight no longer mattered. It took me reprograming my mindset, many years of personal growth work and seeing a counselor to know that even though my marriage ended, it had nothing to do with my weight. Even though I felt like a failure, it was not my weight that was defining me.

I want to tell you right now; you are so *MUCH MORE* than the weight or the number that shows on the scale. Two years ago, I threw my scale away. I decided that it was too much for me to know what the number was. It wasn't even knowing as much as it was allowing the scale to define me.

Like I said, I was waking up and getting dressed to find out what that number said. It got to the point where before I would go to bed, I would just jump on the scale again just to check to see what kind of day I was having. It didn't matter if I knew that I had a good food day or a good exercise day; I needed to know what that number said. I was obsessed.

I was putting my entire hope and trust in a little battery-operated machine that sat in my bathroom all day long. Half of the time, I didn't ever see the number that I *wanted* to see, and the other half the time, it felt inaccurate because it had gotten moved or the battery was dying, or the window was open—all excuses. Anything slightly different that day would make my scale read a little wonky.

It probably *never* was telling me what I really weighed each day. But every day, sometimes twice a day, I continued to trust in this inanimate object. How often do we do that in our lives, where we allow something else to give us value? Or someone else—someone that doesn't even really know who we are. We enable them to give us value and take our power away!

After I threw away my scale, my whole outlook in the morning changed. I didn't just stick my scale into my trash bin, I actually made my husband take it out of my bathroom and get rid of it. That way, I would not feel tempted to go back and get it. (Isn't it funny how we have to trick ourselves?)

Instead of getting up and feeling disappointed or getting excited about some number on the scale, I now wake up and give myself encouragement. Before I get into the shower each day, I take my clothes off, stand naked in front of my bathroom mirror, and look at myself. (I know, that is totally a little weird, right, because there I am just looking at myself naked in the mirror. But that is what I do). I look at myself and say, "Angela, you are so beautiful! Girl, you are gorgeous!! Those momma marks on your belly, you need to rock those today! Your booty, man, that's fine! Your husband loves it, and it's from all the amazing food he cooks you!" Then, I do a little happy dance, and I get into the shower.

I spend five to ten minutes in my shower, and while I am in there, I get excited. I get excited that I love myself. I get excited that I think I am beautiful. And I get excited about the great day I am going to have. I tell myself that I am going to have a great and abundant day. I tell myself I weigh the perfect amount, and I am so beautiful.

I feel excited because I stopped listening to the lies of what my scale had to say. The only thing that my scale could actually tell me was how much mass I took up on this planet. That's it! That is all that the scale is even telling you. How much mass you are carrying around, nothing more. The scale has no way of knowing that you are an amazing wife, good mom, or fantastic employee. The scale cannot measure who you are as a person—stop giving it so much power!

Remember this: whatever people tell you, whether to your face or behind your back, you hear all their negativity—but you have a choice to listen and believe it, or block it out. Their negative words have nothing to do with you. It has everything to do with *their* insecurities, my dear friend. It is not because you are *less than* beautiful. It is not because you are *less than* everyone else in the room. It is because you *intimidate them*. It is because you frustrate them, and you challenge them. They deep down want to be more like you—but fear holds them back, so they attack you.

## Ring Side Chat

I tell you today, my darlings, stand in your purpose. Stand in front of your mirror and tell yourself you are beautiful. Look into the mirror and say it again and again. I want you to go, right now, today, and say, "I am beautiful!" Go! Go now! Find the features that you love about yourself and fall in love with you.

I know that you might not feel like you have any features that you love or that this is completely silly. I assure you that it isn't. Start with one thing. That is how I got started—one thing. For me, it's my gorgeous blue eyes. That is what I love about myself. For you, it might be your Rockstar hair, your dimple on your cheek, your eyes, your smile, who knows, but I want you to go and figure out the things that you love about yourself—right now!

Start there. Then, day by day, as you are falling more and more and love with you, I want you to find other things you love.

And as for our friend Dolly Dimples, after her near-death experience of a heart attack, she went on to lose 440 pounds. She became a world record holder for the most amount of weight loss. She died when she was eighty-one years old. While I don't know much about the dear Dolly, I do know that she recognized that it was never too late for her to change her life, and I believe that for you also. It's never too late for you to fall in love with yourself. No matter where you are right now, it's not too late for you to make the changes so you can live your best life.

# ··· CHAPTER 2 ···
# Side Show Freaks

WHILE MOST PEOPLE think of current-day circuses with acrobats, jugglers, clowns, and elephants, many circuses of old involved the famous sideshow freak. We have already talked about the fat lady, but what of the other notable oddities—Midgets, bearded ladies, the dog-faced man, and of course, Siamese twins.[1]

Before 1950's, there were no surgeries to separate these con-joined twins safely, so they became an oddity of sorts, on display for all the world to see. One of the most famous sets of twins that toured with PT Barnum was Chang and Eng Bunker.[2] They were known as the original Siamese twins because they were born in Siam.

Their sternum connected Chang and Eng. Together they had to learn how to function, not only as partners but also in a society where they were not considered the norm. From an early age, they had to learn how to live in a world of gawkers, a world of everyone staring at them. And I was no different.

• • •

As a child, I always knew I would be a mother, but I never expected I would be every kind of mother out there. Over the years, I have been in  every category of *motherhood*: from single teen mom, to twin mom, to stepmom, to birth mother, and adoptive mother.

• • •

I was seventeen years old when I got pregnant for the first time. I was in a quasi-committed relationship with my boy-friend. I was not his first choice, and he certainly was not mine. But we had mutual friends; in fact, I had dated two others of his best friends and slept with one of them.

At seventeen, I wanted only to be loved. Like many young teenage girls, the basis of love was sex. I was no exception. I knew how to receive *love* was by sneaking out of my parents' house and meeting my boyfriend for quickies in the backseat of his Oldsmobile.

The summer between my junior and senior year, I worked as a camp counselor at a summer camp for children with dis-abilities. Helping children with special needs really fit into my life. I was good at it. It was like I was being prepared for something in my future, but I wasn't sure what. All I knew was I needed and wanted love.

We were together for five months when I got pregnant—two weeks after I missed my period, the morning sickness set in. On my four-hour break from camp, I drove to the near-est Walmart and bought a pregnancy test. My friends and I drove to the local McDonald's, where I peed on the stick in the bathroom. I was hoping my fears would be wrong.

One line. Please one line.

Three minutes later, two pink lines showed my fate.

Pregnant.

When I told my boyfriend that I was pregnant, he replied with, "yeah, so. What-dya want me to do about it? Marry you?"

> Three minutes later, two pink lines showed my fate.

That was not exactly the response I was expecting, but something, anything, would have been more helpful than that. I spent the next month puking my guts out every morning at the camp where I worked. I knew I would have to inform my mother at any moment. I could not just keep that *tiny* fact hidden from her. And then one unlucky day for me, I got injured at work. Because I was under 18 years old, I knew that my mother would find out I was pregnant when we had to go for an exam and an x-ray.

I told her. "I'm pregnant. I am keeping it." Just like that. There was no other question about it. I had claimed my life and responsibility right there. While I was having my injury checked out, we got a prescription for some pre-natal vitamins and a follow-up exam.

When the summer was over, I went back to high school, pregnant. I was one of five other teen moms in my class. I spent my senior year sticking to myself, with a small group of friends, my on-again-off-again boyfriend, and working. My son Taylor was born 11 days after my 18th birthday.

My boyfriend and I tried to *play house* together while I lived at home with my parents. However, we knew that we were all wrong for each other. As the next few months wore on, we knew that we could not continue in the relationship because we did not even like each other most of the time.

After I graduated high school, I went to college for a half-semester. I had a new boyfriend and continued to lead a somewhat destructive lifestyle and left me longing to be loved. I learned early on that babies do not love you back. My son was needy, cried a lot, and certainly didn't care how lonely his 18-year-old mother was. I was a terrible mother. I often left my son with my parents to work, go to college, and see my boyfriend. It was really that last part that made me terrible—always wanting my own needs met. I am thankful every day that my parents were there and able to take care of him the way I could not.

I only completed half of the college semester. One day I decided to skip class and see my boyfriend, who lived an hour away. On the way back to work, I blacked out at the wheel. My car crossed the center line, and I hit a semi-truck head-on in a collision in my Dodge Neon. Thankfully, after the jaws of life and an ambulance ride, I only sustained minor injuries to my leg and a few cuts to my face. Every time I see the pictures of my crumpled-up car, I feel grateful to be alive.

You would think that such a life-altering event would change me, but I am sad to say that it did not. I dropped out of college and became a bit of a drifter while my parents continued to raise my son. It was not until I became pregnant again that I changed my life around.

I had a decent job working for a local fast-food franchise. I had been hired to be an assistant manager and felt pretty proud of the life I was making. Then, one night, a friend of mine invited me to a bar and said, "we could have a few drinks." I was only twenty years old and knew that I would not even be able to get into the bar, but she assured me that she could get me in. While I was not much of a drinker, I decided to throw caution to the wind for one night and let my hair down and enjoy myself.

From the moment I stepped into the bar, there was a man that noticed me. I was dressed in black pleather pants, high-heeled boots, and a skimpy shirt with a heart on it that said *loved*. I was naïve enough to believe I was just there to drink with my friend. I had low self-esteem and knew that I wasn't going home with anyone. He started buying my drinks after my friend bought me my first one. Dr. McGillicuddy's vanilla schnapps with cranberry juice, "a cherry cheesecake," was the drink of the night. The room was spinning when he asked me my age. "I am guessing I am about ten years younger than you," I giggled.

He said, "That would make you twenty-six." And I said, "No, that would make you thirty!" And just like that, he asked me if I wanted to leave the bar and go home with him. It was the first time I had been intoxicated, and I only wanted someone to like me, so of course, I said *yes*.

The next morning, I woke up hungover, naked, and completely confused about where I was. I will never know how my car got parked out front of his house, but it was there. I got dressed and left while my one-night lover lay sleeping. I had no intention of staying any longer than necessary, nor did I ever plan to see him again.

Three weeks later, I found myself once again nauseous and having missed a period. What was I going to do? I kept the news to myself and only shared it with a good friend. I waited to tell everyone else until it was absolutely necessary. The problem began almost instantly. I was sick. Not just normal, run-of-the-mill pregnancy sick, I was puking-every-hour-keep-nothing-down-sick. I was losing weight, there were dark circles under my eyes, and I could barely function.

I told my mother that I was pregnant again, and she told me to make an appointment. The doctor informed me that this kind of sickness sometimes happens to women, but I needed an ultrasound. So just after fifteen weeks of being pregnant, I laid on the exam table where I would see my baby for the first time.

The ultrasound technician made a funny face almost instantly when the image came on the screen. "I will be right back," she said. Moments later, she entered the room with another technician. "See this?" she said to me. I had no idea what I was looking at, but I said, "hum."

"This is baby A, and this is baby B. You are pregnant with twins."

Twins? From a one-night stand? I let that wash over me. I was in a time warp—like a freakshow. My mind was pulled back to the memory of looking at the old displays in the circus. I could smell the popcorn and sawdust. My eyes scanned the collections, and my mind landed on the sideshow freaks of the Siamese twins and an empty display next to them. I knew my face with my twins would have a place right there. That was it. I was now a sideshow freak.

You are pregnant with twins.

As the technician finished the exam, I found myself at a crossroads. I mustered up the strength and gathered words right there. I vowed then that I would change my life and take care of my children. It all changed right there in that exam room. I continued to live with my parents while I was pregnant. If I was feeling unloved prior to this pregnancy, I was certainly at a loss during it. I was twenty years old, with a two-year-old and pregnant with twins, living in my parent's house. The question that repeatedly begged my mind was, *who would want me now?*

I started having contractions one week before my c-section was to be performed. I spent hours at the local hospital before making a trip down to Madison, WI, where they would perform the surgery. I got to the hospital about 9:30 pm when the attending physician told me that 'they don't just do c-sections on demand, or everyone would want them' and then checked to see if I was dilated.

When she realized I was, in fact, dilated, they started to prep me for surgery. I was so tired I could barely keep my eyes open. But just after midnight, two beautiful boys were delivered. Isaac and Jonathon. They made me a twin mom. People used to ask me how I did it, being a twin mom. I would reply with, "I didn't really have a choice." Two babies, whether I planned for them or not. That's how I did it.

I struggled, during that time, wanting to be loved. My self-esteem was non-existent, and I was utterly exhausted caring for three children under three years old. Everyone was always staring at me—freak show! The not so friendly comments kept coming:

"You sure do have your hands full."

"You have three kids, under three?"

"Who's the dad?"

"Where is their father?" Whenever the questions would come, the shame would creep in.

I didn't believe that I was good enough for a husband. I was damaged goods, broken beyond repair. I was carrying the weight of a hundred men, and I often felt like I was the elephant in the room that no one talked about. I heard the quiet whispers, and murmurs about me in my little town— the freak—and the loneliness crept in.

# Ring Side Chat

My dear beloved reader, if you are a single mom, do not give up. I want these words to be for your right now. You are not alone. You did not make a mistake by choosing to have your baby or keeping your baby. You are doing a good job, a really good job.

Nights are hard and mostly lonely, but you are worth so much more than you are telling yourself. I want you to hold your head up high, knowing that you are probably stronger than most because you are doing it alone. Again, I say, *do not* give up. You are not worthless, you are not a bad mom, and this heartache that you are experiencing will *NOT* last forever.

Parenting is hard, and single parenting is exponentially more challenging. Please take time for yourself each day—even five minutes. Lock yourself in your bathroom, if you must! Also, make sure you take a night off without feeling guilty. Let me say that again… without feeling guilt! It's okay to take a break, read a book, take a bath, burn some candles, or even go out occasionally.

You are a phenomenal human, and I am so proud of you for making it this far.

Keep reading. There is light at the end of the tunnel!

I love you!

I believe in you!

# ••• CHAPTER 3 •••

# Strongwoman

GENERALLY SPEAKING, WHEN you think of the strong person in the circus, you think of a man right? However, there were also many famous strong women in the circus. Strength, physical strength of a woman, is really something that many of us don't even think about. Strength is a man's characteristic.

Katie Brumbach (later is her name was Katie Sandwina) was born into the circus life. She was one of fourteen siblings that grew up with performing coursing through her veins. She started performing at the age of two. By the time she was sixteen-years-old, she went by the name of the *Great Sandwina*, and she was undefeated in strongman competitions. After she got married, she began lifting her 165-pound husband over her head with just one hand. She had the strength of an ox.[1]

While her strength is rare, many women possess a power that can overpower anything physically. It is emotional, mental, internal, even spiritual. Every time we choose to not give up, every time we make hard choices, or every time we do something that seems completely impossible, we are demonstrating strength!

For me, I was forced to find strength—a strength at such a young age I didn't even know I possessed. It was the strength to say goodbye. You see, I faced a choice—the most difficult of my life. I gave up my fourth child, my son, Michael, for adoption. I was twenty-one years old.

● ● ●

Have you ever longed for something? Have you ever felt like you are missing something or that you need something—maybe a feeling of emptiness that you need to fill? Well, imagine it. I wanted something more. What did I want? I was unsure. But, I sought after *more* to fill my heart. For me, *more* came in the form of men—men that were not good for me. I ended up getting pregnant again with a man that I met in a bar. I was underage, and someone snuck me into a bar and gave me way too much to drink. I mean, as I relive the story, it shocks me. I met a *much older* man who took me home to his house, we slept together, and I found out a few weeks later that I was pregnant.

What a shock to him that the woman he had only seen twice after that bar room meeting would show up at his work in the middle of the night to say she was pregnant. I didn't even tell him. I just handed him a note across the desk because I couldn't even bear to say the words out loud. His response was, "So what." I blinked, he turned away, and I left.

I faced the pregnancy alone. A few months into the pregnancy at the ultrasound, with my best friend in the room, I found out I was pregnant with twins—a one-night stand and twins. Boy, was I lucky! What are the chances of that? (Yeah, go home and tell that to your family at twenty years old. That is a great time. Not).

When I was seven months pregnant with the twins, I met a man who led me to the Lord. I really just wanted another relationship, and his only goal was to set my heart on fire for Jesus. I remember late one night while we were on the phone, him asking me why I loved myself. I had no real answer. I didn't love myself. I didn't even like myself at that point. I was so broken as a human being, and I felt ugly inside of my soul.

That night, in the middle December, while I talked to this man on the phone, being massively pregnant, I was shown some kindness. This absolute stranger started giving me reasons to love myself. He told me I was a kind person. He loved me. He wanted the best for my life. He told me that I was loved. He told me to never give up. He said he could see that I really wanted a better life for myself—even then. His words cut me to my core, and as I sat sobbing in my bed, I told him that I just wanted a man to love me. And he said, "You don't need a man; you need Jesus."

I had been going to church for years. I knew who Jesus was, but I didn't have an accurate picture of what a relationship with Him would be like. That was the night that I gave over my soul to the One that created me. Now, this would be a really great story if I told you that I fell in love with the man that brought me to the Lord, and we lived happily ever after, the end.

> You don't need a man; you need Jesus.

However, that is not what happened. I will tell you, though, if there are such things as angels, that man named Mitch was one. I only spoke with him a few times after that, until the day my twins were born, and then I never saw him or heard from him again, but the impression of his words went into my core and would surface later in my thirties.

About three weeks after the twins were born, I met my first *was-band*. (I don't like to call them *ex's* because they are valuable as people. They simply are people who once were married to you.) We met online. Now that might seem pretty typical nowadays with all sorts of dating apps like *Tinder*, *Plenty of Fish* and *E-Harmony*, but that was not the case in the year 2000. We had *Yahoo Chat!* and that was the extent of how people met online. You would pick a *room*, with a topic you were most interested in, and then you would jump in on the conversation. Following the discussion, the private messages would start amongst the people you met.

On one particular day, I got into a private message with my then *was-band* who was looking for a church. At that point, I had become very involved in going to church any time the doors were open, so I offered him a few dates that we could get together. There was an upcoming pizza social on a Friday night. I invited and welcomed him to my church. He lived fairly close, and I wasn't interested in dating anyone, so it seemed okay to ask him.

It was a pretty small church, without many single people—but for me. I was *the single* person in the church—with three kids, mind you. When a new man came into the church, it often seemed like fresh meat amongst the old ladies who wanted to see me settle down. I had a lot of people tell me that "it made sense for us to get together," and besides, "who was really going to date a single mom with three kids out of wedlock anyways?"

If you can see here what was being said to me, you can understand why I struggled with my own value. I didn't see myself as attractive. I certainly didn't have any qualities that were going to attract a man to me—except the fact that I was incredibly able to bear children. I listened to what people said, and I believed them.

"I had better jump at the chance to be with someone who was only a few years older than me and had a great job."

"He would be able to take care of us."

"He was a Christian after all." Well, that sounds like a match made in heaven.

My *was-band* and I went out on our official first date on my 21st birthday. We went out to dinner with another couple from my church. I no longer trusted myself alone with anybody from the opposite sex, seeing as my track record was not all that good. I really wanted to do *everything right* in this relationship. I wanted to prove my worth. I was significantly skewed in my thinking of what dating should look like. I had read books about people waiting until their wedding day for them to kiss. And I truly wanted that. Finally, I wanted to be *the good Christian girl* after being so wrong for so long.

In trying to do everything right, I am able to look back now and see how wrong my thinking was in all of that. We were on the *fast track* to getting married. In fact, we married in September, just six months after my birthday. Because I am so incredibly fertile, conception was not even slightly an issue. I got pregnant on the honeymoon, and then, we came home from our three-day honeymoon to *play house*.

Two weeks after the honeymoon, things changed. First, I found out I was pregnant—which was exciting for about one hot second. My *was-band* worked long hours, and then when he came home from work, he was incredibly controlling. It's highly possible that he had controlling behaviors before we were married, but I was unwilling to notice that detail. (I was blinded by love and desperation). None the less, after a series of events, he broke a lot of items in the house, and then he pulled a knife out of the butcher block, and pointed it at me. I thought he might seriously hurt me or even snap and kill me! Our eyes locked, mine in fear, his in rage. That moment was suspended in time. It was at that time that I could have lost this fight. However, something in the heat of the moment broke—he left.

• • •

I was alone, battered, abused, no self-worth, pregnant, and twenty-one years old. I spent a lot of time in prayer. I felt let down. I felt angry. How could this God I loved *so* much leave me like this? I couldn't understand why I got pregnant again.

I laid in bed night after night and prayed the Lord would change the situation. I am not proud to admit that I begged God to let me fall down the stairs so I would no longer be pregnant. I didn't really want that; however, I was such a mess mentally, emotionally, and spiritually. I knew that I was not capable of caring for another child.

At that moment, I wasn't even working. I had to find a way to sustain us. My *was-band* had left, and now I was barely functioning and keeping food on the table. In fact, until I got a job, I was borrowing money from people, accepting donations from the church, and the local food pantry, just so we could eat.

I was praying for an answer—any answer—and an answer came, not as I expected.

One day, I had gotten home late. I was taking a couple of night classes at the local community college. My dad was sitting in my living room, watching my children, who were asleep. He said to me, "Angela, I need to talk to you about something." He took a deep breath and looked at me. "I think that you need to give this baby up for adoption." He paused. His voice faltered and cracked, but he pushed on. "There is a couple in the church that has been wanting a baby for a long time, and they can't bear children, so I think that you should give him up. We would never ask you to give up the other kids, but we really feel that this is the right thing to do."

My stomach lurched and seemed to fall to my feet. I immediately felt sick inside. I felt myself falling, or that I was no longer standing—or something—and I had a knee-jerk reaction. "Absolutely not! No way! Not my baby!" How could I give a child up for adoption? What would people think of me? What would *my child* think of me when he grew older? Would he know how much I loved him? Would he understand?

My dad left my house. I was crazed with anger, and I went to bed. That night, I laid awake most of the night tossing and turning. And then, I started to pray. I asked the Lord to give me a real tangible sign that this was what I should do. What came back to me was kind of bizarre to me, but I was told that I should go and talk to someone. The pastor's wife.

Now the pastor's wife was the sweetest lady on the planet. She had an open-door policy, and I loved her. She was the woman that always welcomed you in, to sit down and to drink a cup of tea or coffee. I went to her house, and I prayed the whole way there. I begged God to tell me in that next hour what I should do. "Don't sugar coat it, God, I need answers, and I need answers now."

I got to her house and she welcomed me in. We sat there on her couch. I grieved my marriage. I told her how much I was hurting. We talked about options. I told her what my dad had said to me, how angry I was, and how I didn't think I could ever just give away my own flesh and blood.

After I had laid it all out for her, she looked very distraught. And when I asked her what was wrong, she told me that she didn't want to tell me because she didn't want to weigh on my decision. I knew what I had prayed, and I knew that I was there seeking answers, so I begged her to tell me. She said, "Oh Angie," (that's what they called me) "Just one week ago another couple came to us and said, what if Angie's baby is the answer to that couple's prayers. What if God's plan for them includes her?"

I knew as the words were leaving her mouth that I had my answer. I knew that I was going to give my child, that I was carrying, up for adoption. The answer settled into my heart in a profound burning way. I knew what I was going to do.

My *was-band* had already left the state, but I had to find the strength to call him with this news. Where was I going to find that strength? I prayed. You see, he was getting ready to enter into a divorce agreement with me, but I still needed to tell him.

I mustered as much strength as possible, and I told him that I thought we should give up our baby for adoption. Silence. I told him he would probably never see our child since he had already moved a thousand miles away from us. Silence. I told him I felt this was the right thing to do. Silence. I hung up that call, waiting to see what his answer would be. After a few days, he called me back and let me know that he had agreed to the decision. That was it. Our baby was going to be raised by another family.

●  ●  ●

Now, I needed to tell the couple. How was I going to find the strength for that? I prayed. The pastor and I set a time for the meeting. It was a bit of an ambush, honestly. We met at my pastor's house, arranged by my pastor, but they weren't given any details of what this meeting would be about. They knew that I would be there, but that was about it. The meeting started. I sat down with them and told them what I was facing. They nodded and looked at each other and then back at me, and they looked at the pastor. They had empathy in their eyes. After finishing my story of how I came to be in this situation, I asked them if they wanted to adopt my baby boy.

Stunned, yet with hopeful smiles they looked at me. Silence and peace filled the room—well, gasps really. Their eyes filled with tears and confirmation. I sat across from them giving them the answer to their prayer. God sure knows what he is doing. They were very excited. They told me that they wanted a few days to think and to pray, but they really thought that it was going to be the right decision for them.

After a few days, they called me to tell me that they wanted the baby that I was carrying. I spent the next several months doing life as a single mom, trying to figure out how I was going to raise the three other children I had. It wasn't like in the movies where the birth family and the adoptive family spend every minute preparing and going to the doctor appointments together. Granted, we did a few things together, but mostly I was alone.

I went back to college to try and better myself and I worked part time. I was trying to hold everything together, all while being pregnant and raising three children under three years old. It was not easy. It was a bit like a three-ring circus. In fact, acts were going on in every ring. I never quite knew which direction to watch. I was constantly juggling work, school, children, and the incomprehensible loneliness that my soul felt. My growing belly was a constant reminder of every failure I had ever experienced and every wrong choice that led me here. Yet, it also reminded me that I was delivering a miracle to a family who would care for him the way I couldn't.

● ● ●

The day came for me to have Michael—that was the name that his adoptive parents picked. I always wanted what they wanted. So he was always Michael to me, even when I was pregnant.

We got to the hospital early in the morning because I had to have a cesarean due to prior c-sections. I spent four days in the hospital with my baby, Michael. It was heartbreaking and joyful for me. Joyful, very joyful, but also devastatingly heartbreaking.

At one point, the entire adoptive family (cousins, aunts, grandma, and grandpa) were all coming up to visit with their new baby Michael, just down the hallway from my room. I gave them permission because I knew that it was vital for them to bond with their baby. They were laughing and telling jokes, being so incredibly cheerful, at the same time that my heart was breaking, just down the hallway. He was to be their first baby. AND he was supposed to be *my first* baby that my *was-band* and I had together. However, that wasn't the plan for me.

I was discharged from the hospital four days later, and I stayed with the pastor and his wife for a week during my recovery time. I couldn't face my children. The very thought that I would have to look into my precious babies faces knowing that I gave away their brother was killing me. I felt like I was wrongfully harming my kids by taking away their big brother opportunities. The twins would not get the chance to have a baby brother, and I felt so sad that I was doing that to them. I felt like I was betraying my children.

During my recovery, I stayed with the pastor and his wife. I was able to hear a story from a woman who was attending our church. She was about eighty years old, and she told me that she had given a child up for adoption about sixty years earlier. She told me that no one ever knew she had placed a baby for adoption. My breath caught. No one? She gave me a look of love. She thought that her story would bring me comfort—to know that she could survive and make it through the grief. Her story gave me great peace in knowing that she chose to share this secret with me and also the burden she had been carrying for so long. I appreciated her wisdom and her grace.

At the end of the week, I went home to my babies. A few days later, the adoption hearing happened. I sat in the courtroom, alone, and then on the stand as if I was a criminal. The judge repeatedly asked me if I understood what I was doing.

If I knew the ramifications of the adoption? Did I understand that I was voluntarily giving up my rights?

His blunt words left me feeling so cold, so dirty, so ugly. I was despondent through it all—numb! I answered the questions, feeling that this was an out-of-body experience occurring simultaneously. I said all the right things.

"Yes, I am voluntarily giving him away."

"No, I am not being paid any sum of money from the adoptive parents."

"No one was forcing me to make this choice."

"Yes, I understand my rights will be terminated." But inside, my heart was splitting in a million pieces, and I felt dead.

As my last words fell from my lips, the court hearing was over. I can't even tell you what was said other than his new parents were able to pick up Michael from foster care. (The state required a short waiting period). I knew they were anxious to bring him home. I hugged them, and I whispered in his mother's ear, "go get your son."

I fled from the courtroom! I ran as fast as I could out of the building. I did not want to linger or talk to them or anyone else. I just wanted to get home and crawl into my bed and cry as fast I could. With the covers encasing my body, I cried, and I cried. I cried so hard that my body ached, my throat was raw, and I could barely see out of my eyes.

Finally, I was all cried out—empty, hollow. But time was still ticking, so I picked myself up that afternoon, and I drove numbly to the day care to pick up my other children. It had started to rain, steady and heavy. I remember thinking to myself how fitting it was—God was crying right along with me. When I picked up my kids, my son asked, "mommy, are you sad?" To which I replied, "yeah baby, a little." I couldn't explain to my three-year-old what was going on. The rain continued to pour as I was driving. With wipers whipping back and forth, I shouted, "Really God? Can't you just make it stop?"

And suddenly, the rain stopped. The sun started peeking through the clouds, and a rainbow appeared in the sky. I pulled my car over to the side of the road and got out of the car. My eyes beheld, not one rainbow in the sky—but two. It was as if God was giving me a sign of His promises: a promise for Michael that he would thrive in his new family and a promise for me that I would be okay. A promise that I was strong enough to give up Michael for adoption.

● ● ●

Michael turned 18 a few months back. I have had minimal contact with his family throughout the years. I have always known he was okay. I knew his grandparents, aunts, and uncles. If I ever inquired of Michael, they were sure to tell me that he was well.

For his 18th birthday, I sent him a letter telling him that I was proud of him and loved him. I sent a second letter to his parents, thanking them for raising such an incredible human being. With the two letters, I gave Michael the wedding rings from his biological dad and me.

Over the years of my life, there were a few times that I was extremely poor—almost destitute. On those occasions, I would have conversations with my parents about how I would pay my bills. They would suggest that I sell the rings; however, I always stood my ground about those rings. They were the one thing that connected me to him, to his life, and to all things that were right in my world.

A few days after his birthday, he reached out to me on social media. We had a few brief interchanges, and then he asked me whether I would like to meet with him. My heart was delighted. We arranged to meet one afternoon at a local park. It was raining again, and I remembered that day so long ago—the day where I was given a faithful promise that God would carry me through the most challenging moments of my life and give me strength.

When I walked up and saw him standing there, my heart was in my throat. This tiny baby that I carried for nine months was a man. A man who looked so much like my other children, and yet, had the face of my *was-band*, except his eyes—his eyes were mine. His eyes were crisp and blue and filled with life. We spent three hours talking the afternoon away. And then, it was time for us to say good-bye. I asked him if I could hug him. To which he nodded.

For one brief moment, I held that man in my arms and was transported back eighteen years to the hospital room. To a time when I knew that all would be well and he was the most precious gift I could have ever given to another person. We said our good-byes and headed to our cars. I drove three blocks away and pulled over, and cried. I thanked God for allowing me to see Michael, hold him, and let him know how much he was loved.

## Ringside Chat

Like many women who have placed their children up for adoption, I spent years carrying around shame and guilt about the decision. While many say or think that adoption is a noble thing, and it is, there is an overwhelming grief and ache of sadness that can take a toll on a person's heart and mind.

If you are one of these women who has placed your child for adoption for someone else raise, I want first to commend you. I know you might be thinking that you are nothing special, but you are—you truly are. It takes a lot of courage and strength to go through nine months of carrying a child. It takes even more strength to take a deep breath and place that child you carried in your womb into the arms of another to raise.

There is an aching and longing in your soul that cannot quite be explained into words. For many, it causes deep devastation that can be difficult to recover from. And if this you, my dear one, I have been there. I want you to know you are deeply loved. While that might be hard to hear, it is the truth. The gift you have given to your son or daughter is meaningful and will not be left unnoticed.

It does not mean that you are less than worthy of a good life; in fact, quite the contrary. You gave another family an extraordinary gift because you did what you thought was best for your child. And that, my dear friend, is the *strongest and most noble thing* you could have ever done. Do not give up. Hold your head up, knowing that you are the reason another family was given such a precious child and a chance to be a family. You are the reason for someone else's joy.

● ● ●

Maybe you think there is no relevance here for you in this chapter. You may not know what it's like to give a child up for adoption. If you never have, then you are absolutely right. You don't know. However, have you ever given up on a dream?

Have you ever felt grief when you gave up those dreams? Have you experienced the *what ifs* again and again? Have you ever traded joy for shame, blame, and guilt over a decision that happened too long ago for you even fully to remember how you got to this place? While it is not the same circumstances, I would challenge you to look at why you are blaming yourself for something you felt you had to do. Stop carrying around the bags of shame that don't prove you are any stronger of a person.

The real strength comes when you find forgiveness for yourself and the joy to know that you have done the best that you knew how at that moment. Hang on, my dear friend. You may not know the answers, and you may not see the outcome for many years. Like me, you may have to wait eighteen years to see promises fulfilled, but I assure you, they will come! Be strong while you wait.

I love you and believe in you.

# ··· CHAPTER 4 ···
## The Illusionist

ONE OF MY absolute favorite acts at the circus is magic or illusion performances. One act, in particular, is called the metamorphosis. The illusionist and his assistant come onto the stage, with a variety of props. The theatrical show is all about how the magician gets handcuffed, bound, and locked into a trunk. The assistant takes a beautiful covering (which looks like a fancy sheet), stands on top of the locked box, and raises and lowers the sheet, and then counts to three. One. She lowers the sheet, and you can see her face. Two. She lowers the sheet again, and you can see her face. Then, three! She drops the sheet, and in a blink of an eye, the illusionist is standing on the box, with the assistant nowhere to be seen.

The illusionist does quick work to show that the woman who was his assistant is locked safely in the trunk. The audience applauds and everyone stands in wonder how this trick is done. I have no idea how the trick works, but that is just it! It is a simple illusion—a sleight of hand. Illusions make us believe that something truly magical is happening when it is nothing more than a lie.

I spent an entire marriage living much like the illusionist's assistant—working hard to shed a good light on my *was-band* and yet, always falling short. Why? Because the assistant is not the one in the limelight. It's still about the illusionist—always working to make him look good.

Early on in my second marriage, I struggled with the issues that we had. I was twenty-four when we got married, and my second husband was thirty-eight. I lived in depression and poverty after giving Michael up for adoption, and I honestly was unsure how I would make it in the world.

I had met my second husband, also on the internet, not believing that I could do any better than him. We eventually got married—eloped to Vegas. I only told three people that I was going to get married. Looking back, I knew the reason I eloped was that I didn't want anyone to talk me out of it. I was ashamed of the choices I was making, but I was so desperate for someone—anyone— to love me that I eloped.

I flew out to Phoenix, and we immediately drove to Las Vegas. We got married at the Hollywood wedding chapel, with only the employees of the chapel for witnesses. That same night we drove back from Vegas to his house in Phoenix. We were both broke and couldn't even afford to stay for one night there. The first time my husband saw me naked was when I changed my clothes in the car on the five-hour car ride back to his house. It wasn't romantic. It wasn't exciting. And I felt ashamed of my life.

Those two weeks were the sum of our entire relationship. I didn't know much about him or his life other than what he had told me, and most of the things I learned later were a lie. I flew back home alone at the end of our honeymoon. About a month later, he drove all that he owned in his Ford Taurus north to Wisconsin, where we started our life together in my small two-bedroom pest-infested apartment.

At the time, I had been providing for my family as the general manager at a local ice cream franchise. I had always dreamed of owning an ice cream shop and had even gone to franchise school in hopes that I would someday be the owner of the company I worked for. I loved what I did, but the hours were long and filled with stress. We often fought about me working and him staying home with my children. He often told me that he felt emasculated by me and that I was not a good wife by working outside the home. Eventually, I realized that our relationship would never work if I did not let him take the lead.

So, I did. One Sunday morning, I walked into work, put my keys in the safe, and quit my job. I was reckless! I had my three small boys at home and now no real income. However, I desperately wanted to be a good wife and Christian. The sermons being preached at my church repetitively were "the man should be the head of the household." The man *should* work, and the wife should stay home. The very same statements that my husband was making to me. Because I wanted to be a *good wife*, I submitted. I gave up my dreams and became a housewife.

● ● ●

For a while, our marriage was *okay* at best. I pretended that I liked football, cars, and all of the things that my *was-band* enjoyed. He would go to work while I did the best job I could at home—being a mother to my three boys. After the first year of being married, he convinced me that we should homeschool our children, so, like an obedient wife, I did what he asked though entirely unqualified.

We had moved into a slightly better house than my dump of an apartment, and I was able to make the best out of what I had to work with. However, I was no teacher. I constantly felt like I was in over my head, and I had no clue what I was doing. I was *uneducated*. I didn't really know how to cook a proper meal, and I often found myself depressed due to the traumas I had experienced earlier in my life.

I had been hoping and praying that I would get pregnant, even though I knew there was very little chance of that happening. When we first got together, he had told me the possibilities were slim to none, of me bearing a child with him, but all I heard was, *there is a chance.* I was stubborn, depressed, and often defeated. (Eventually, we went on to adopt children, which you'll read all about in chapter five).

Everywhere I went, and week after week I would act as though I was happy. That was my job. To act as a good little wife. And, internally, I felt miserable. I found myself often alone at church with my kids, while my *was-band* was conveniently working or too tired to attend with me. I would put on the best smile that I could muster and share with anyone who inquired about him the truth—that he was working—or give some little white lie about "how he didn't feel well and needed to rest." I constantly made excuses for him. I constantly tried to be the magician's assistant by making HIM look good. The truth was, he was a fraud… and so was I.

Looking back, I struggle to remember if any part of our *church-going* was authentic when we went together. I knew that I loved God, but I will never know if my *was-band* did. I often found myself on the circles' outer edge that I longed to be a part of at church because I was caught in this *pleasing of others* game.

I served in every capacity that I knew in the church. When the church was open, I was there. I often found myself there mid-week, checking out a book from the church's small library or praying in the sanctuary. If something was happening, I was there. I was always the woman in the third pew, hands raised, desperate to love the God who I knew and to be the wife that everyone said I should be.

But I wasn't. No matter how hard I tried, I wasn't. My life was a lie—right down to one of the final Facebook posts

I made about my *was-band*. We had been fighting for years, and honestly, I knew that things were not good. We had made a final last-ditch effort to make it work for six weeks leading up to the demise of our relationship, but it was not working.

Our marriage was in peril, but my now *was-band* decided to leave for a ten-day trip to Arizona. I had begged him not to go—that he should stay and continue to work on our relationship—but he still left. He wanted to visit his mother. She and his sister had bought him a ticket to go for a visit just after Christmas. I was not invited.

I knew we weren't going to last much longer, but I continue to pretend that everything was fine. I continued to do what *good Christian wives* do and turned my head to all the problems we had. I felt shamed repeatedly into believing that the marriage I was currently stuck in, was the way marriages were.

I spent those ten days while he was gone trying to make sense of our relationship. There were no nightly phone calls to check-in. There was just him doing whatever it was he was doing and having the time of his life. I stayed behind, once again, and held down the fort: I cared for the kids, I worried about the money, and cleaned the house. Alone.

I thought about the last seven years of my life and what I had learned in church. I had heard teachings that were twisted and made me want to scream, but it was right there in black and white. Husbands had complete control of their wives. It was perfectly acceptable for name-calling, berating, and occasionally for a violent exchange to occur—wives should submit.

And so, I did—over and over and over again believing if I just got a little thinner, if I offered more sex to my husband, or if I just cleaned the house a little better, then we would be *just fine*. I did all of that, and we weren't *just fine*. We were the opposite of whatever *just fine* was.

I had been turning a blind eye to the abuse for years: to the pornography, the unexplained late-night outings, the money frequently being gone, the barrage of name-calling. The names I would never even call my worst enemy. I turned my eye to it all, believing I was being *a good wife.*

*It was perfectly acceptable for name-calling, berating and occasionally for a violent exchange to occur—wives should submit.*

And then the night happened. The night that I wrote the biggest lie I ever had on Facebook. I made a post saying, "Yay. I am so glad my hubby is coming home tonight!" But I wasn't glad. I wrote it because I felt expected to write it. I wrote what I thought the world of Facebook would want to hear. I was keeping with the illusion that everything was fine and dandy.

By the time I had written the post, I was feeling incredibly ill. On the way to the airport to pick him up, I had a migraine so bad I was vomiting on the side of the road, and I was in the midst of a full-blown anxiety attack. Seeing him walk towards the car I felt such conflict and the anxiety attack worsened. He put his stuff in the car, sat in the front seat, and did not show any concern for my health. He didn't care, and he did not even thank me for picking him up.

My *was-band* slept on the couch that night after an argument in the car. The next day we had another fight that would finally end our relationship. He was angry about various things, and so was I. Very violent and physical exchanges occurred in the heat of that night. I was minutes away from calling 9-1-1 when I told him that he needed to leave. His suitcase had still been by the front door.

And he did leave.

For the first time in almost eight years, I had peace. I was able to breathe. He walked out of the front door with his suitcase in hand, and I leaned my back against the door. My marriage was over. I didn't have to live the illusion any longer. I no longer needed to pretend that everything was okay because I knew it wasn't. But, I was also finally free.

Weeks later, after the announcement of our separation, I was shamed into believing I was a terrible person, a terrible wife—even worse—a terrible Christian. I was told I should stay together at all cost and beg him to repair our marriage.

I didn't. I could no longer live with myself and believe that I was not worth more than just being the *magician's assistant*. I stood my ground. I watched my world fall apart. And I lost almost everything. However, I gained freedom that day. I gained the independence of knowing that I did not have to live in a lie. I did not have to be abused anymore. I did not have to carry the burdens of shame continually.

And neither do you.

## Ringside Chat

Moms, wives, women: you are better than a hurtful life. You are worth *so much more* than the shame you carry. You are not the shame that was placed on you by someone else.

Let that go. (I have tools and ways to do it—I want to help).

Forgive yourself, my dear one.

You can have a peaceful life filled with joy, but you HAVE to stop blaming yourself. You have to stop shaming yourself into thinking you are not valuable—because you are!

You are so much more than someone's assistant; you are the Ringmaster to your own show. You are the one in charge of leading your life. You do not have to live a lie, no matter how hard it is. You are worth so much more than that.

If you are in a situation right now that looked like mine, please get help to get out. I spent too long believing that there was no hope for me—that God would not love me if I left the situation. That God would somehow stop loving me if I was divorced. God *DOES LOVE* you and will be there even if those around you leave you. It won't be easy at first, but you deserve to have a life filled with peace, love, and joy.

Also, my dear ones, I am here for you. If you need an ear, email me. My email address is choosetoday366@gmail.com. I will be here for you.

I love you. I believe in you.

# ••• CHAPTER 5 •••
# Birthing an Elephant

HAVE YOU EVER seen an elephant up close? I'm not talking about like at a zoo from behind a cage and hundreds and hundreds of yards away. I'm talking about up close and personal with an elephant. Maybe you haven't. I'm probably one of the fortunate few that have seen an elephant regularly and up close. I live in a circus city, and therefore, we have three elephants that come to our town every summer and spend the entire summer in our community. Visiting the circus, I get to see these beautiful, gentle pachyderms weekly.[1] They are the largest land mammal on our planet, and they should be revered, and it is with such great joy that I'm able to look into their gorgeous eyes. I have pet their trunks, and I have ridden on these giant creatures.

The thing about elephants is they are pregnant for nineteen to twenty-two months.[2] As a mom who's ever been pregnant, I'm sure that you have never wanted to be pregnant for twenty-two months. By my fifth month, I was somewhat annoyed by the whole growing a baby, and by eight months, I would be like, "get this kid out of me!"

I know that I never wanted to be pregnant as long as an elephant, and yet, in a way, I experienced a twenty-two-month process that brought two more children into my life. How? Did I have back-to-back pregnancies? No, not exactly. I went through a fostering and adoption journey that was a LOT like birthing an elephant. Now I didn't have to carry an extra 250 pounds like an elephant, although the stress that I endured did pack on a couple of extra pounds.

• • •

When I was married to my second *was-band*, we had my three boys, but we had really wanted to have children together, and I fought for a very long time against the idea that we could not have kids. It devastated me that, month after month, I would get my period. I would be sad because I wasn't pregnant. I knew deep down in my heart of hearts that my *was-band* would not be able to give me children.

When we got together, he had told me we never would be able to get pregnant—99% confirmed for sure; however, I clung to hope that there was a 1% possibility that we could. And when we finally didn't, after about three years into our marriage, I knew that we were not supposed to have children together. I finally gave up the notion that I was ever going to get pregnant with him and be content with the children we had.

• • •

One day while we were sitting and watching television, an advertisement came on about foster care. It had the cutest little blonde hair, blue-eyed girl I'd ever seen. My then-husband looked over at me, grabbed my hand, and said, "we have to find a way to have children."

My heart stopped in that instant because I had resolved to believe that we would never have children together. We would have our three boys, we would live happily ever after, and that would be the end of it. But suddenly there he was telling me, getting my hopes up, that we should find a way to have kids—invitro, foster, or adopt, anything for kids.

I took what he said to heart and ran with it. The very next day, I was on the internet looking for ways to bring children into our lives. I searched and searched. I researched *in vitro fertilization*, sperm donors, and many other different medical procedures. Everything I saw was going to take a *lot* more money than we had. But I was desperate to find a way. I thought if we could just have a child that we shared, it could bring us together and enhance our marriage—even save our marriage.

Remember, I was broken. I was carrying around deep hurt and anger from giving up Michael for adoption, and I thought that a child would fix that hole for me. That gaping hole seemed to have created a cavern between me and my *was-band*. I ignored the brokenness, and I pressed on towards the goal of bringing a child into our home.

I looked up adoption, which I already knew plenty about, but never on the side that I would be the adopter. I called agency after agency and was told the same thing repeatedly. Adoption costs money. The exact words from one agency explained if "I was looking for a *perfect white baby*, it would cost me approximately $25,000." We definitely did not have that kind of money. In fact, we had very little money at all. I thought there had to be a different way.

I spent all of my free time looking at the registry for adoptable children, even knowing we didn't have the money to adopt. I came across two little girls who were available and called and spoke with the social worker. I had illusions of grandeur that I would hop in the car and have them home by dinner. I was quite delusional at that point. A charming social worker quickly corrected my imagination. However, she did not leave me hopeless. If I was serious about adoption with minimal cost, she told me that we should become foster parents.

• • •

With a deep breath, I looked up foster care. I looked up all these different avenues so that we could have kids together. We finally settled on becoming foster parents, and I thought the process would take a month or two for us to become licensed. Then we would have the kids—a little baby that we could share and delight in. We would never want anything again.

I wanted a baby girl, and I thought for sure we would have her. We would rock, kiss, and help her sleep—all would be well with the world. However, one month turned into two, which turned into four, which turned into eight. Why the delay? Why no little baby? It was the procedure and hoop-jumping of the foster care system. We soon found ourselves performing in the *Foster Care System* act. It took over one year to become licensed.

Why? There was one delay after another for paperwork reasons. Many times, the agency had a high rate of turn over—social workers quitting, and our case changing hands. It was all about the timing. One year later, as we sat in the training office, I asked the person who was giving us our license, what it took to be a foster parent, and how children came into foster care? She responded with, "some children are abused who enter the system; and then they are taken back to their home and abused repeatedly. The county is ready to pull the kids out in a minute, and then other kids come into care out of nowhere."

I felt so mixed up inside. The system she was explaining felt like chaos—a circus—but *without* enjoying the show. My thoughts were racing:

*What if we get a call and there are two children to immediately care for?*

*What if it is a whole family?*

*What if there isn't a baby but an 11-year-old to care for?*

I had to put my fears aside and step into this completely. We were licensed on November 1st. I remember thinking *this is it. It's time for us to get our little baby girl and bring her home.* That's what I had told the foster care agency that I wanted. It was in my heart. I was going to add a baby girl to our family. I was not going to do anything other than that. I had three boys. I always wanted a little girl.

Yes, I am guilty of dreaming of having a baby girl—someone I could dress the same as me. Instead of playing dolls and having a matched set, we would be the matched set—my miniature me. I waited and waited for the phone call to come in. About a week after we became licensed, I got the call I had been waiting for from the agency.

They called to tell me that they had two children who were in the foster care system, a girl who was eight and a boy who was five. Siblings. Wait… I was confused because I had asked for a little girl under three years old. That's what I wanted, but the licenser assured me that these two children were the right kids for me. Two? Wait, two? Deep breath! *Ok, I* thought, *I can do this. I'm a mother of twins. This is just like that—I think, yes. Ok. I will meet them.*

We met at the local zoo, which was right near my house. I walked through the gate and headed over towards our meeting place. Immediately I saw the social worker and two red-headed children. The girl, Amber, had a haircut that looked like somebody had taken a machete and cut off her a ponytail. It was ragged and rigid, but she had these beautiful green eyes. She could barely walk. She dragged her foot behind her. She was overweight and in a pair of pink sweatpants. Her brother, Joe, had broken front teeth that were black and dirty looking. He was in a blue sweatsuit that matched his sisters. His hair was a mess, and his eyes hung down. He didn't speak.

Here they were. Two children who looked disheveled, beaten and broken. I'm ashamed to admit this, but they were not very cute. They weren't even Cabbage-Patch kid, cute. They were just not cute at all. I wanted to run. I wanted to cry, yet my heart was breaking.

Do you see how sometimes we set an image in our mind, and when reality hits us, we fall apart? We think, *this can't be right because it doesn't meet our dreams or expectations.* (Mine is usually followed up with that ugly cry). But maybe, just maybe, we have to take a chance and see what we can do with the circumstances given to us.

> I'm ashamed to admit this, but they were not very cute.

I wondered to myself how I would ever take care of these children. I was so stuck on their outward appearance—I didn't even think they were adorable. This was not my idea of a picture-perfect family. When I sat down and talked to my husband that night, he asked me what I thought of the kids. I said, "I don't know how I can do it. I don't know how I can care for these two children who don't speak, can barely walk, and are both in diapers. They are eight and five. They're not what I wanted, and they're not even cute." And as I said it, I laughed and cried because I wasn't even sure what I was doing. I know it's raw and ragged, but that's the truth of it.

With a deep breath, I took them for a weekend—respite, they called it. I promised the social worker I would give them a chance. That very weekend, these two children that had been tortured and abused by their birth mom got to experience something different—something new!

We went for a walk downtown. I was told again and again that Amber and Joe would not lead *normal* lives. They would probably not ever walk normally. They would be in diapers forever and they would never carry on a conversation. And more than likely, never be able to read. And yet, these children and I walked downtown enjoying a lovely November day in Wisconsin.

We visited Santa and sang Christmas carols to the best of their ability. We took a carriage ride around the square. We enjoyed the beginning of the holiday season—complete with hot chocolate and marshmallows. There were smiles. There was laughter. It was then that I realized that there was something special about these children. It was then that I realized that they were so much more than what people could see about them. I saw them!

I agreed to take them on.

Taking on two foster children along with my own three birth children was anything but easy. Remember how long an elephant is pregnant? I carried the burden of going to social worker visits and going to home visits with their birth mother. I didn't like dealing with the system that was broken that required my children see their birth mom every week, sometimes twice a week, all the way until the day of termination of her rights.

My children had to go through weekly regression—five steps forward with me, and fifteen steps backward with her. Amber and Joe were subjected to verbal, physical, and emotional abuse again and again. The system takes children and gives them days of hope, food, and love, and then an afternoon going back to the abusive treatment the system is trying to help them get out of. What kind of sick circus is that? It's one that lasted twenty-two months for us.

There wasn't a honeymoon period where you find out that you're pregnant, and you get to have this baby. No—foster parenting is much more like carrying and birthing an elephant. You are hoping for nine months and end up in it for nineteen to twenty-two. You carry this weight on your shoulders and wonder every day if these children will be forced back to their birth mom. I wondered if these children were ever going to call me mom. I wondered if they would ever get past the trauma, the heartache, the downright sadness of what their lives were, and if they'd ever move on.

Again, the process was nineteen months before we were able to go to the courthouse and have the birth mom's rights terminated and my foster children to become my adoptive children. How does all of that happen—the rights of their mom have to be terminated? Think about that for a minute. Her rights would be taken away, and I would assume full responsibility. That in itself was a birthing process.

Moms, you know how painful labor and the birth process is, and to terminate rights is usually a five-to-six-month journey. However, the birth mom's termination of rights took our family almost nineteen months to complete. We had to show the court enough evidence that these two sweet children were never going back to the abuse.

Ok ladies! Who is ready for a three-day labor? Yes, to top off a nineteen-month pregnancy with a seventy-two-hour labor is a circus! But in the scope of things, three days in court to terminate rights is pretty much unheard of anywhere—especially in the state of Wisconsin.

● ● ●

The day of court came. It's like that feeling—my water broke! Everything that you as a mom are looking forward to, from holding your baby to watching them grow up, is happening right now. We think that labor will be a few hours, maybe a day at the longest, but for us, it was a three-day labor-intensive birth (of sorts).

I had to be sequestered, away from the trial, while witness after witness testified to the abuse my foster children had repeatedly endured. That was like feeling every contraction without seeing the result or any progress. It's like all the nurses have the information, and I was just confined to my bed waiting for the doctor to come in and tell me that it was time to push. That is how the trial felt.

Finally, the time came (just like from labor to transition) I was able to testify. YES! (Think of labor—this is that moment of prep time). I am ready to push (so to speak). I sat in the courtroom, and I gave testimony to how good my children were doing (push). How I cared for them by meeting them where they were developmentally, not where others thought they should be (push). I knew I could help them reach their potential because I started where they were and set an expectation for them (push!).

Following my testimony, the social worker began to speak (this is like hearing another mom down the hallway in the hospital screaming and pushing. You know the pain she is going through, but it's out of your hands).

The social worker testified about the first time she met my-soon-to-be-daughter—how she didn't speak, was only wearing a pair of underwear, and had eaten a cold hot dog right in front of her with m& m's put-on top (think more screaming and pushing).

The social worker testified how her birth mom sat off to the side (as she watched Amber eat) and claimed that she was old enough to feed herself and make healthy choices for herself. She testified about Joe. The abuse and pain that he suffered at the care of his mother. The social worker also testified about the very first time that she had ever laid eyes on my children. Their skin was so pale she wasn't ever sure that they would get color or pigment from being outside. They had never been allowed to play outside! They had been under their birth mother's care—abusive care—what an oxymoron!

I listened, watched, and could feel the fear and pain well up inside me—just like real labor while all of this was happening. Remember this "birth" had been going on for three days. As the social workers' words came to a close, it was now in the hands of the judge. Right. This is that moment when the doctor comes in, and we are in full trust that *the delivery* will be the outcome we are all waiting for.

The testimonies, the evidence, the painful stories had all been discussed. Now it was up to the judge to terminate the birth mom's rights. The clock that had started ticking three days ago, was ticking even louder now—tick, tick, tick, tick. The judge returned from his chambers, and I could not read his face. I wasn't sure if it was going to be good news or not! He swept over everything— read and reread a few papers. Finally, he looked up. It was as if I was just to give that final last push and then the flashback of the water breaking three days ago, the pain, the contractions, the pacing, lots of anguish and anxiety, and more pain and the final push—relief!

Suddenly it was over. Just like that, the judge looked at my *was-band* and me and awarded us full custodial rights to these two children that had been in my care for almost twenty-two months. It was over. They were ours; we had endured the pregnancy, the labor/delivery, and the birthing process. It truly was like birthing an elephant.

## Ringside Chat

Oofta! It takes a lot to birth an elephant, and I am not jealous of those pachyderms for even a second. Here we are on another adoption story, and this time, I found myself on the receiving end. The receiving end of joy. But not without a lot of hardship and work. That is the crux of it all, my dear one.

I will tell you that fostering and adopting has been another of the hardest things I have ever done. Yet, the most rewarding at the same time. It was not easy. The chaos that often ensued in my life was a daily struggle. I found myself daily fighting against a system that was/is broken and trying to speak life into two children who were equally as broken.

I am not going to sit here and tell you that it was easy, or that even after the termination took place, that everything was popcorn and cotton candy. That would be an utter lie. The termination of the birth mom's rights happened nine years ago. There are days when things in my household are still affected by my children's life in their birth home.

We have had to work through long-lasting effects of trauma and abuse, while continuing to push forward at the same time. There have been multiple therapists, mental health situations and even calls for the police to come to our home as our children have gotten older. My children suffered deeply in their birth home, but after they came into my life, they learned the art of living and *enjoying the show* through the learning process.

They have made fantastic progress and achievements. My daughter Amber graduated highschool, learned how to play the saxophone and is off to college, studying culinary arts at a school for adults with disabilities. My son Joe, who still struggles daily with an Autism diagnosis (believed to be brought on from the abuse and trauma he suffered), has just started on the high school track team. Twelve years ago, I was told these children would never walk, talk, and lead normal lives, and now our normal looks like the sky is the limit!

After you birth an elephant, you don't just stop. The birthing might be over, but then you take on the challenge of raising the elephant you just gave birth to. Think about a 250-pound wobbly creature that doesn't know how to use its limbs. That is often how life is. Trying to figure out what will work and how to find joy through all of it. Even in the hard stuff.

That's what life is about, my dear ones. Joy takes work.

Joy is a daily burden—the proof that you are deciding to live. That's it. You get to choose how joyful your life is or how hard you want to make the labor of that project you are trying to birth. I am sure you have heard the saying, it's a labor of love. Many people refer to their jobs, their lives, or some other demanding projects as such—just like birthing an elephant—a labor of love.

● ● ●

What labor are you going through right now that might need a push? Are you stuck in a life that leaves you feeling unhappy? Maybe it's time to look for a new career. Push, push, push.

Is your marriage falling apart around you? Do you find yourself disappointed with your love life? If so, maybe it's time to talk to someone about your relationship, talk to each other, or try counseling? Push, push, push.

Maybe you are just wondering how you got to age thirty-five and still want more out of life. Stop and look around you. You are at the circus—the circus of your life! It is all around you, with chaos ensuing at every corner, and you just want something more. This is the time, my dear ones, to give your life a BIG push in a different direction.

It will not be easy to birth the elephant we call *life*, but the joy that comes after will be worth it. I promise.

You are loved, and I am here for you.

# ··· CHAPTER 6 ···
# Put on a Happy Face

CLOWNS, YOU EITHER love them, and they are one of your favorite parts of the circus, or you hate them because you think they are creepy and weird. Usually, in this scenario, there is no in-between. I am not here to change your mind in any way about the feelings that clowns bring you, but I would like you to imagine for a moment that you do, in fact, like clowns. For some of you, I understand that this might be a stretch.

Clowns offer a few different things in the circus. The first thing that they bring to the table is comedic relief. One of my favorite kinds of clowning is slapstick comedy. Often, a clown will do something nonsensical, and then another clown will end up slapping the first clown. It ends up in a sort of dance between the two with slapping, stepping on each other's over-sized shoes, and falling to the ground. Eventually, the two clowns will come to an "agreement" of sorts, and they will shake hands, and then the scene will be over. The entire event is used to create laughter amongst the audience. The bigger the fall, the more laughter created.

Another reason the circus needs clowns is to create a break in the show. Maybe there was an aerialist high in the air, and the next act requires some setup; the clown or clowns will come rushing out on the stage to provide a short bit of laughter before the next act.

The clowns were my most favorite act as a child and still are to this day. When I was growing up, there was a show before the Big Top show, called "Put on a Happy Face." A gentleman known as Jimmy Williams or Happy the Clown, would greet the children at the door and then lead them into an arena. There would be a table with a mirror with light bulbs around the outer edge, some makeup, brushes, and a mannequin head with a red wig on a small stage. Directly behind him, hanging on a coat rack was a clown costume.

He would introduce himself and then get to work transforming his face into a clown. He was patient and kind as he answered questions about why he was putting his make-up on a certain way, and he would throw jokes in along the way. Right before our very eyes, we would see a transformation into a completely different character, but really, he was Jimmy Williams, pretending to be *Happy the Clown*. Afterward, he would lead a group of parents and children down to the Big Top, where we would get to be first in line for the show.[1]

> That's what life is really about—creating joy, even when things seem ridiculous and completely out of control.

Clowns bring a certain amount of controlled chaos to the party. To the audience, their performance may seem entirely out of control and utter pandemonium. But the fact is, the clowns have rehearsed and rehearsed their act. They know how to hit each other without getting hurt, they have practiced falling, and they have perfected many of the gags that people see. They bring joy out of the chaos.[2]

That's what life is really about—creating joy, even when things seem ridiculous and completely out of control. When my first *was-band* left me, I had made a post on Facebook talking about how I was feeling. Someone sent me a message privately and chastised me for *acting* happy. The thing was, *I actually was happy*! I had made a mental note that I was no longer going to be miserable with the time I had left on earth. My JOY was in jeopardy if I continued to live miserably.

When my second *was-band* left me, I decided how I was going to handle life from now on—with Joy! Now, it wasn't easy. More than once, I hit a place of darkness, and I wasn't sure I would recover from it. One day, I had a friend of mine tell me that I needed to *work on myself*.

I had no idea what she was even talking about—*work on yourself*? Did she want me to go to some huggy-feely talking seminar or something, where we would all sit around and sing kumbaya? I was not interested. I didn't realize that working on myself meant so much more than what she was implying.

● ● ●

One afternoon, my life hit the point of rock bottom. Everything was falling apart after my second marriage ended. I was indeed on the verge of losing everything when I decided that something had to give. I was frustrated at myself for the kind of mom that I was to my kids. My children deserved so much more than I was able to give. I was frustrated because my house was always a mess. And there never seemed to be enough money to make ends meet. I felt like I was in a taffy machine being pulled in every which direction, sure to snap at any moment.

I remembered my friend telling me about *working on myself*, so I looked at the email she sent me. She had invited me to a conference—a seminar of sorts. I made a choice. I would go to my friend's crazy seminar and check it out. It was the first decision in a million decisions that set me on a path to something more. The take-aways from that seminar are more than I could ever fit into this chapter, however, the biggest one was this: I needed to stop allowing the *chaos to steal my joy.* I was the keeper of my joy. Me. Only me.

I had been playing *the victim* in my life for far too long, and it was time to stop. I spent so much time blaming my *was-bands* for nearly all the failures in my life. After all, I thought, *they were the reason that I was in this situation with so much misery*—my blame game? My *was-bands* were creeps, they never sent me child support, had affairs on me, etc. But the truth was, I carried around a lot of scars—a lot of baggage. I had to give Michael up for adoption—I was still reeling from that decision even ten years later, and the negative voices never seemed to stop listing all my problems end in my head.

Listening to the words at the seminar, I realized I was allowing the negative experiences, voices, and feelings to control my joy. I was giving someone else the power and control by running these negative thoughts in my head. I had expected to find happiness or joy in others. No, more like I was expecting *them* to make me happy! When they couldn't, then I was the victim. Wait! Wait! Hang-on, it just clicked! Right there at that conference, I had an epiphany.

*I was not a victim unless I chose to be a victim.* I was responsible for finding my own happiness—for making my own joy. It was up to me—not anyone else. I sat in that chair in the middle of the conference room as if time had stopped for a few minutes while I let all of that new information sink in. It was true. I felt it. I was capable of making myself happy—of finding joy. I had to stop making excuses. I had to decide, be a victim of chaos or find victory in joy.

My mind started quickly making a list:

1. The reason that I had so many kids, and so little money, was all on me. I was perfectly capable of working. I could get a better job if I wanted to. My children were my responsibility and no one else's. It didn't matter if my children's fathers were in their lives or not; that was on them. I could choose what kind of mother I was going to be.
2. I was not a victim when I gave Michael up for adoption. Rather, I made a choice. The conscious effort to give a child a better life when I knew I could not care for him.
3. The reason that my house was always a mess, again, that fell on my shoulders. I could make decisions to change that. I could teach my children to help me with chores. I could also learn more about staying organized. I could stay up an extra 30 minutes doing the dishes, sweeping, and mopping. I could decide to get rid of the clutter. Me, all me.
4. The reason I was miserable was that I was waiting for others to make me happy. I could choose to stop trying to find my value in other people. I could know my worth and find joy—just because I wanted to be happy. It was time for me to stop accepting mediocre and truly go after what I wanted in life. It was time for me to stop being a victim.

I came home from that weekend with a purpose. It was the pivotal moment in my life where I sought to change—not only because of the seminar but also because I wanted so much more out of life. I had been beating myself up for years over the chaos I encountered in my life, and I never entirely accepted the responsibility for it. I was making excuses one after another about the things that happened in my life.

As I was driving home, my mind flashed to a comment one of my children made after my second *was-band* left. "Now, we will never get to go to Disneyworld." I remembered questioning my son more about that, and he told me he felt that way because he knew I was a single mom—a single mom with five kids. My children also all knew how poor we had been when I was married. Now, we would be even further behind.

In my son's mind, the divorce meant that we were destitute, and we would never go to Disney. That was a piece of hope he had been holding onto, and now it was gone. When I was married, I had promised the children we'd go to Disney. The plan had always been that once Joe was tall enough to ride the rides, we would go. We were guessing that Joe would have to be about ten years old for that to happen. He was nine at the time of my divorce.

Does that paint the picture for you? I had this conversation with my children weeks before the conference. While I was sitting in my car leaving the meeting, reflecting on what the speakers said about *taking control of our lives* and replaying "Now we will never get to Disney," I had a powerful idea. I wondered to myself, *what would I have to do in my life for me to take my children to Disneyworld by the time Joe was tall enough to go?*

● ● ●

When I got home from the conference with a renewed sense of purpose, I made a plan. I talked with my parents about my desire to go to Disneyworld. They shared with me that they wanted to go to Disney as well. They were turning sixty the following year and had never been.

At the time, I knew that the only way for me to make my children's dream of heading to *the happiest place on earth* come true was to get a second job. I currently was working for myself, running a local lady's athletic gym with one of my best friends. But if I wanted to create a dream vacation, I would have to work for it. What was I going to do with my children because hiring a babysitter was out of the question because it would defeat the purpose of saving money if I had to turn around and pay someone to watch my children?

With this desire in my heart and me taking action, two weeks later, someone posted online about a job. The request and details of the part-time job were posted on social media. A couple was running a local motel who were looking for someone to watch the front desk. This couple was preparing to have their second baby. The perks of the job were that children were welcome to tag along! I applied for the job and was hired immediately.

My children had no idea that I was working the extra hours to save for a Disney dream vacation. But I was. Every extra dollar I made went into a savings account. Within a few months of diligent saving, I had enough money saved for our tickets. The plan was for me to surprise my children on Christmas morning.

It was the first Christmas in years that I was single, yet my house was filled with joy and laughter. My parents had bought each of my children their luggage, and I bought us all Disney-themed t-shirts. I had the kids unwrap each of their presents and try to guess if they could see any pattern amongst the gifts. Finally, Amber said, "I think we are going somewhere, maybe?" in a question of confusion.

And then Taylor screams, "WE ARE GOING TO DISNEY!!!!! BEST CHRISTMAS EVER!"

I still remember the tears that fell from my face as we all put on our Disney t-shirts and lined up in front of my fireplace. Mine had a picture of a glass slipper that read, "She lived happily ever after," and I felt those words deep within my soul.

A month later, my five children, parents, and brother boarded a plane to Florida. The week was filled with all kinds of magic. When we had gotten to Disney, we were given special passes because of Amber's and Joe's disabilities. We were able to skip the lines with fast passes. We had so much fun riding roller coasters, one after another. Taylor tried out for American Idol, which felt like his greatest dreams coming true, and we went to the most incredible shows.

One of the most iconic shows at Disney is the Indiana Jones-themed show. During that show, they called for volunteers, and it was exciting because I got chosen! People were chosen from all over the audience, and when I found myself on stage, a man in front of me turned around, and there was my brother standing on stage as well. And we both broke out into great laughter. We were choosing joy in every moment—every moment.

I was able to see that no matter the circumstance, there is still joy no matter the heartache. Like a group of clowns driving into the arena in a tiny car, the joy began to fill my heart, and that is where you can find joy as well.

## Ringside Chat

Are you reading this right now, feeling frustrated by life and feeling like I wouldn't understand what you have had to face? Well, you are right. I will never be in your shoes, similarly that you will never walk around in mine. However, I can understand that you may not have had an easy life. You may have been divorced, or experienced loss, and grief, unforgiveness, similar to me. You may have had a horrible childhood or experienced the pain of an abusive marriage. Whatever the situation, my dear one, I empathize with you. You do not have to stay this way. There is always a choice. The choice starts in your head and ends in your heart.

There is more to life than just being miserable and going through the motions. Once you can take a step back from whatever you are facing, accept what is, and the responsibilities you played in this life, you can choose to live differently.

Once you decide to accept your life, you can THEN CHOOSE JOY whatever the circumstance of chaos is. Once you have decided to have joy, then you can make a change for something different. Maybe you can go after the job you always wanted, plan a vacation you have always dreamed of, or even simply decide to no longer live-in misery. It comes down to more than pretending. It is putting on a happy face and deciding to become someone who is the essence of joy—someone like a clown.

I hope you can find some joy today, my darlings. I love you so much and believe in you.

# ••• CHAPTER 7 •••
# The Ringmaster

EVERY GOOD CIRCUS show starts with a phenomenal Ringmaster. I have been fortunate enough to see Ringmasters that are the most incredible singers and performers on the planet. Some would even call the Ringmasters the *stars of the show*. I beg to differ. The Ringmaster is the *glue* that holds the show together.

If you have ever watched the Ringmaster throughout the show, you can see what I am talking about. The Ringmaster is dazzling and helps to keep the show flowing. He is also standing guard to make sure that everything runs in perfect harmony. He is much like a mother hen to her chicks, then the star.

The Ringmaster is the one that introduces each act. He will give you a dazzling bit of information about the performer and then directs your eyes to which ring that person is performing in.

"Look there, the beautiful acrobats on the high wire."

"Here come the elephants."

"Send in the clowns."

He is in charge of showing the audience where to look and where not to look.

And then, while the most death-defying acts are being performed, the Ringmaster stands and waits with the rest of the audience. I have watched as there have been near-mishaps and have seen the look of concern on the Ringmaster's face, right along with the rest of us viewers. And then, moments later, a smile, knowing there is reassurance as everything with the performer is all right.

I once asked the Ringmaster from my local circus, how many mini-heart attacks he has in a single day watching the performances of so many death-defying feats. He replied, "too many to talk about, but I will always watch and care for my people."

That's it! Right there! That is the epitome of living, of parenting, and of running and operating our own lives. I believe we are the Ringmaster of our lives. We are the glue that holds our own shows together.

Think about this a minute, if you will. Just like the Ringmaster, there are many things that are outside of your control. You can guide, direct, even plea with those in your lives to do the right thing, or do the things you want them to do, but ultimately, the choice is up to them. Just like the Ringmaster can point out where the audience should look, he cannot control what is happening with the performance. He simply must wait and watch and see how the show plays out.

You cannot control what your husband does, what your children do, or even your best friend's choices. They each have the ability to make their own choices, even if you can see they are going to fall flat on their face.

● ● ●

When my son was eighteen years old, he decided to move out of the house. Now mind you, he did this two weeks after his birthday even though he was still in high school. He wanted to be independent. Over and over again, I would watch him as he would make mistakes in so many things. It broke my heart. I knew that there was nothing I could do to change his mind.

I would pick him up after work, and we would go for a drive, and I would beg him and plead with him to change his mind about his decision. He would stand firm and tell me he was an adult and wanted to make the mistakes on his own. It was then, I realized that I had to let it go, and whatever the outcome, I would be there for him.

It is not easy to watch someone fall flat on their face, but it is the Ringmaster's job to stand to the side and let the performers do their act. In the same way, we cannot control what people do around us.

Standing and watching the performers is not the only job of the Ringmaster. There is another important job that is required. The Ringmaster must make the hard choice when to cut an act out of the show. Maybe an act is not working in the spot where it currently is, so it needs rearranging. Or the music and the flow of the act is not working right. Or an even bigger issue could be a personality clash between performers. Someone with *diva syndrome,* perhaps. Where they have to have everything just so, and then throw fits of anguish when it is not exactly what they want. Maybe they complain too much, or their act isn't good enough yet, and they need to keep practicing.

These are all very good reasons for a Ringmaster to cut a performer from the show or rearrange for a better performance.

You can do the same thing—rearrange your show, so things work better. Maybe that means that you are over-whelmed on a day-to-day basis because something isn't working with your schedule and it is time for you to say *no.*

Perhaps you are trying to please too many people out of fear of lack of belonging. Or maybe, just maybe, you are trying to hang on to control when really, it's chaos.

I have found that people often forget it is absolutely okay to say *no* to things in their life that don't serve them—from activities and people in their lives.

I once had a friend who complained every time we spoke. If it is was sunny outside, she would say it was too hot. If it was rainy, then she wished it was sunny. Her kids were always getting on her nerves, and don't even get me started on what she would say about her husband. On and on it went like this, and after a while, I would find myself sucked into the same trap. I would find myself irritable and complaining about the exact same things, even when there wasn't anything wrong!

I would come away from friend dates with her feeling the exhaustion of being overwhelmed and usually grumpy. What I realized was it was time for me to take control of my life. I needed to give myself permission to cut that woman out of my life.

I knew if I really wanted my life to be the *happiest place on earth*, and a place I did not want to escape from, but rather too, I would need to take back control and truly become the Ringmaster in my life. It meant that I had to sit down and look at my schedule. It meant I had to look at my friends' list, my finances, and who and what I was investing my time in.

It's easy just to live your life on auto pilot and do the next thing mindlessly. It's when you stop and take control of the things you can control; you are able to make the changes you need.

Becoming the Ringmaster of my own life also meant for me, getting divorced. It meant taking back the control that I had given away to someone else and allowing them to rule me.

I am not saying in any way that if you have a bad marriage, you should automatically get divorced. Please hear me out on this. I am saying that you do not have to live your life being abused, made to feel small, or go unnoticed.

You get to decide what your life is, and only you get to choose. Being the Ringmaster means you determine who is in your show and who is not. The ones who are in your life because they have to be: your family, your employer, your co-worker, etc., only have to be apart of your life as much as you let them be. The same goes for the others around you.

> I am saying that you do not have to live your life being abused, made to feel small, or go unnoticed.

## Ringside Chat

This realization came to me incredibly unexpectedly, the reverse of me being a Ringmaster to my own life. At thirty years old, I had a best friend. We had been best friends for eight years. We had children near the same age, we hung out together, and our husbands hung out together. Then I went through a divorce, and suddenly, my best friend and I were no longer in sync with each other.

I loved this woman more than anything—more than any other person I had ever been friends with. I hung out at her place all the time. When I was going through a tough time in my life financially, and I couldn't afford to buy groceries, I would go to her house to *shop* for groceries. My friend would give me food! She would say, "here I have this extra pot roast in the freezer; you take it, feed those babies." I would do the same for her! When her family was taking on tough times, she would come over and tell me that she wasn't sure what she was going to do about dinner, and I would load her up.

That was just the way our friendship was. She went through breast cancer, and I was there. I was there with her when she shaved her head. I was there with her through several treatments. We went shopping together. We did a breast cancer 5k together. I was there when she told me that she might not be capable of having other children after the treatments. I had been at the hospital hours after she had several of her babies, and I couldn't even imagine her not being able to have any more. She was an amazing mom, and I loved her so much. We were the best of friends.

You can imagine how very devastating it was for me when I got the letter in the mail from her that said, "I am sorry, I just can't be friends with you anymore. I don't understand your life anymore. I don't understand you. I don't understand what you are going through. We are just too different now. I think it is time to part ways."

I was devastated—crushed beyond all existence. I cried for days and I grieved the loss of my best friend as if it was a death. It hurt for a long time. Even now, there are occasional twinges of pain when I wish I could call her. Every time I drive past her old house, I still think of her.

She was the Ringmaster to her own life! She decided what act to cut, and unfortunately, that act was me.

After that, I wasn't sure if I wanted to make friends with other women. And so, I mourned the loss of not only my *was-band* but also my best friend. But then, one day, I met a woman. We started developing a friendship. We kind of, sunk into each other, in a way that was awkward at first, like many friendships begin. I was guarded. But she understood me, and she became someone that I could bounce ideas off of. We were able to enjoy each other's company. We laughed together. It took a long time, but now, she is one of my close friends. I consider her to be in my circus.

I, also, have a few other women in my life that I can talk to. I go to them when I am sad and when I am angry, and I am frustrated with my children. When I can't speak to anyone else, I go to these women. I found solace in these women when times have been tough—like when I almost bankrupted my business. I was doing so poorly financially that I had to take out loans from a few of my friends and family members—it was humbling, rough, but they were there for me.

I have celebrated birthdays, new babies, promotions, and other exciting times. They were the people I went to when I found out I was going to remarry. And they cheered and showed up when I decided that I would have a flash mob wedding in the center of my town on a Monday night in the freezing cold. They were there.

They were my circus. They were my tribe of misfits that I had chosen. The acts that I decided to put back into the show! So many times, the Ringmaster will cut and replace acts. The same is with life. It is ever-changing. The great thing is you get to decide!

You decide what you will keep and what you will cut. As long as you choose to be the Ringmaster of your own life, your show will be incredible. Remember, the option is solely yours—accept it and own the part!

Don't ever be afraid, dear one, to cut out the acts that are toxic and abusive. Those kinds of acts, will not serve you in life. Whether that is a spouse, a family member, a job, or even a good friend. Make sure the people and acts you allow in your life will bring you joy. I am here for you if you need an ear or someone to talk with. Just send me an email: chooseto-day366@gmail.com.

I love you, and I believe in you!

# ··· CHAPTER 8 ···
# Juggling the Chaos

SINCE I DECIDED to be the Ringmaster in my life, I would love to say that my life has been a fairytale ever since, but that would not be true. The difference between where I was twenty years ago to where I am today is, I have learned to be a better juggler.

●●●

When you watch jugglers, it's easy to stand in awe as they move from two to three to six balls. And then they light some batons on fire. After that, chainsaws. Who doesn't love a good juggler with three to five chainsaws? As their finale, they attempt something even crazier, like being blindfolded, juggling chainsaws while riding a unicycle, or something else incredibly daring.

The thing is, I get excited watching a juggler when he just is tossing three or four balls because it is something that I know that I am not skilled at. And, I have since learned that no juggler starts with chainsaws! That would be completely ridiculous. They start with one ball back and forth, back and forth, then two, and then three. As they get good at three, they move on to something else to juggle.[1]

Life is the same way. We can't do what we don't know how to do. I could not love, forgive, or even live a peaceful life until I learned how to do those things.

● ● ●

After my divorce and my great epiphany on life, many things happened, and I changed. People asked me how I made such significant changes and told them. I had to dream again! I created a dream board or a vision board.

If you don't know what that is, I will give you a brief synopsis. You create a giant board with pictures of what you want your life to look like. Sounds simple enough, right? It really is that easy! Once the images are up, you believe you can have what is there on the board. There are thousands of books out there about people who have created their lives, by starting with pictures in their heads. Have you ever heard the saying, "thoughts become things?" That is really what a vision board is.

The first vision board I made was honestly not *a board* at all. I found some pictures that I wanted, or things that I desired and set them to a slide show on my phone, and added a song I liked. Several times a day, I would look at my pictures. There was a wedding ring, a Disney trip, pictures of money, and some other things. Within the year, I had all of the items in my photographs. How? My conscious mind kept these dreams in focus in my subconscious mind, and therefore, my thoughts became my action. You are what you focus on and about.

Over the years, I have gone on to create several more vision boards. I have put things like dresses, flowers, appliances, trips, and even a Starbucks symbol on my board. Now don't get too excited because I do not own a Starbucks, however, I am the proud owner of a Starbucks coffee maker! Sometimes you just need to be more specific, I guess.

• • •

Just after I created my first vision board, I started to date again. A part of me wanted to meet the man of my dreams—I knew he was out there. I wanted someone who was the popcorn to my cotton candy, someone who could bring me some balance, and organization to my chaos. I had been filling out online dating apps and received plenty of emails. It was like my emails were chum to all of the *fish* that I was attracting.

No, maybe not chum, but more like shark bait. I mean, I was a promising catch, after all. Divorced twice, five kids in tow, any man would be lucky to have me. Feel free to insert an eye-roll here, as I did. For a year and a half, I watched, waited, and looked at my vision board with high hopes that eventually I would find a husband that could join me in my *happily- ever- after* life.

I knew exactly the kind of man I wanted, and I refused to settle for anything less. Date after miserable date, I would see if the prospect was to be someone who would join my circus.

One day, I got an email from a man who told me he wanted to go out with me. I didn't like his picture, and frankly, was uninterested. However, he kept asking. Little did I know, he had seen me several times around the community and was already head over heels for me. If I would just accept a date with him, in his mind, we could all have our happily ever after.

I refused. For three months, I refused to go out with him. Then one day, when I realized that I was never going to get him to leave me alone, I told him that I would give him one hour of my time—a date at a local bar where we could shoot some darts or play a game of pool. I figured the second he saw how bad I was at these games; we would be done.

When I walked into the bar, however, something else happened. I met the man that felt like the best friend I had been missing for my whole life. In one instant, my heart was gone and was sitting with the stranger that wouldn't leave me alone. He had two daughters and I had five kids. Together there were nine of us, and I, along with everyone else I knew, thought we were crazy. He asked me to marry him after twelve days of being together. I said yes. The ring was the exact ring that I had put on my vision board a year earlier.

For five years, we remained unmarried. We lived together, and we even had a baby named Eli; we were living a remarkable and beautiful life. (If any of you are trying to keep up, yes, that means we have eight kids together—a perfect 10, and still unmarried).

> He asked me to marry him after twelve days of being together. I said yes.

Part of me was not ready to be married. I knew what my faith said about not being married, but I was also profoundly scarred when it came to husbands. Do you blame me?

And then it happened. One day, my best girlfriend asked me flat out, "why we didn't get married?" I had no honest answer. I was ready to fire off a ton of excuses, but I didn't. I thought about my sweet man and all the times we had talked and talked about getting married, but the details just couldn't be panned out. We were trapped in a never-ending cycle of who to invite, where to have the ceremony, and who would be in the wedding?

Meanwhile, we were juggling kids, the house, tragedies like fires, and starting our own businesses. A wedding did not seem like a top priority—no matter how much we wanted to be married. We just weren't married.

In January of 2018, when I usually am crafting and creating what I want to put on my vison board for the following year, I thought, *what the heck? Why not?* And I stuck a picture of a bride and a groom on my dream board.

On March 11th, my beloved came into our business and looked at me and said, "Hey babe, how fast do you think we could get married. I am tired of *not* being married." I didn't know if he was serious or not, so I said something like, "well, three or four days for the courthouse, but we don't have all of the kids this weekend, so maybe Monday?"

And just like that, a plan was formed. We decided to have a *flash-mob* wedding on the courthouse steps on March 19th. I wore a white 1950's style dress, with polka-dotted hearts all over it. All of our kids were there. We exchanged ring pops and then danced to Bruno Mars afterward. The whole thing took about fifteen minutes. When it was all said and done, we drove over to the local Mexican restaurant with everyone that showed up and ate chips and salsa and drank margaritas. I could not have had a better wedding. I stopped all of the pressure of following a plan that wasn't mine. I stopped trying to juggle chainsaws when I was only qualified and equipped to juggle handkerchiefs.

## Ringside Chat

Ladies, the *things* in life—the things we are constantly pressuring ourselves to do: to meet someone else's expectation, and for what? For their praise and opinion of you? Are you still trying to be popular and be a part of their club? Think about it. Would meeting their expectations really change the way they feel about you? No, it would be another failed event because no matter what you do, *they always move the bar*—that something has to look a certain way, or it has to be perfect. Ladies, it doesn't.

Life can be whatever you imagine it to be. Even if it feels like a circus.

I don't want you to think that my life is always a hardship or always sunshine and roses. It's a mix of both. It is good and bad together—not all of one, and none of the other.

I'm going to be blunt here; marriage takes work. I'm speaking to that. To be clear, I am not a marriage counselor, or count as "an expert" (obviously as I have three marriages under my belt). However, I actually AM an expert. . . BECAUSE I have three marriages under my belt.

My husband Edward and I don't always get it right, but there are a few things that we *do* get right.

Our saying is, "You can't build a new house with old broken bricks." That means you cannot stay living in the past with your hurt and shame—a house built on broken bricks will crumble the same way a marriage will crumble if you do not protect it and live in the now. We work hard to let go of grudges, shame, or things that have happened in the past. We stay focused on the now.

The second thing is we continue to work together to show each other our love. We have read books, studied relationships, and learned about who the other person truly is. My husband and I read the book *Five Love Languages*, by Gary Chapman, and took the principles of the book to heart. My husband knows that my primary love languages are *acts of service* and *gifts*. Every year for Christmas, my husband works very hard at picking out something super special for me (usually jewelry) and tries to show me how much he loves me by the gifts he purchases. Acts of service: my husband cooks daily and cleans the house—I know I am loved!

Any guess as to what my husband's love language is? Physical touch. Yes, that is right, my husband likes sex. What man doesn't? Like many couples in relationships, we had *the fight*—how much sex? When do we have sex? Why only sex? Here's the fight. I'm busy juggling the chaos and need to get the crap done, and he needs some play time— with me. Can't he see the giant to-do list? Hello? Well, I would say no, and he can't and is wanting more. It never seemed like we could quite get the timing right of when to have sex, and it was the source of constant arguing.

The more I talk to women about this topic, the more I realized that I was not alone. Well that's good, but what is the solution? How can my husband and I work through this constant argument? As a mom, I am sure you can understand what I am talking about; remember *the look* I referred to at the beginning of this book? So, how did we deal with *the look*?

Ladies, I will let you in on our marital secret. We made an agreement—a sex agreement. We sat down and had an open and honest conversation about how many times a week we were going to have sex and what days. It was a bit of a nego- tiation really. It behooves me to tell you that in my house, we have sex—a lot—five days a week. (You might not want to share *my details* with your husband). However, the fighting about sex has completely stopped.

Here's why. There is no longer confusion as to when *it* is going to happen. I know that may not seem romantic or get your vibe going, but it works. I know what nights of the week we are going to be making love, and he knows what nights we are not. He also knows not to ask on those nights, which gives me room to breathe. We also, in our agreement, have made room for some other negotiations, such as, maybe we are going to have a little more sex on a particular day of the week (Sexy Sundays), and so we will negotiate not to have sex a different day, so I (and my vagina) can get some rest.

Ladies, here is what I know: your life is what you make it—even the intimate parts of your life as you juggle the chaos. Remember, you don't have to struggle with juggling chainsaws every day. You can take it easy and be happy with a few handkerchiefs. It's all about how you see it that matters. No matter the struggles you are facing, the balls you are juggling, know that you can do it with joy—it's your choice!

I love you, and I believe in you.

# ••• CHAPTER 9 •••
# The Day the Clown Cried

THE YEAR WAS 1944. The date July 6th, just two days after the country was celebrating the joy of independence. I can only imagine the times back then. You could see the wear and tear on the country and yet hope amongst the people. There was sacrifice and hardship, but there was also a little fun in the midst of that—it's circus time!

Think about the joy it would be if you were fortunate enough to go to the circus—the circus in 1944! In the good-old-days, a person would put on their *Sunday best* and spend the day enjoying all of the sights and the sounds of the Big Top.

Even back then, the tents were made of canvas and striped the iconic red and white. The difference, though, back then, compared to my sweet tent that is put up each year in my little circus town, is the size. Back in the 1940s, the Ringling

Brothers had a tent that could hold up to 9,000 people! As giant as a large stadium, complete with three rings!

The circus had traveled to Hartford, Connecticut, July 5, 1944. But, before the circus was to open that day, an unfortunate thing happened. The circus train was delayed. Many circus folks believed it to be a bad omen—missing a show. Even though the evening show on the night of the 5th still took place, people were worried.

And then, on this particular Thursday afternoon, July 6th, the band could be heard playing "Stars and Stripes Forever." While this may seem patriotic to some, it was the song that meant there was distress in the ring. A fire had started in the back corner of the ring, inside of the menagerie. The band was signaling to the rest of the circus that there was trouble.

The Ringmaster tried to lead the people out of the tent, calmly and orderly, but the tent soon lost power, and chaos ensued. More than 160 people died that day, and over 700 people were injured. Many animals died tragically due to the fire because they were trapped right where it had started. A picture was captured during the unfortunate event, and it spread across to the local newspapers. The world-famous Emmet Kelly, a tramp clown, carrying a bucket of water to douse the flames. The newspapers deemed that tragic day, *The Day the Clowns Cried.*[1]

And a sad day it was—losing everything—digging your way through rubble and chaos. I have been there.

Twice in my life, I have experienced a fire—earth-shattering, devastating fires.

● ● ●

The first was a crisp night in April. I was sitting in Eli's bedroom, trying to get him to go back to sleep for the third time that night. I was nursing him and checking out my usual social media accounts, wondering if anyone else was awake in the middle of the night as I was when I smelled just the faintness waft of smoke.

I sent my husband a text asking him if that was smoke I was smelling. We had a beautiful fireplace that we often used to partially heat our house during the cooler months of the year, and this particular evening was no exception.

I heard my husband leave our room, and then the next thing I heard him say was, "Fire! Get the kids out now!" I jumped to my feet and sprang into action. Most of the children slept in their bedrooms at the top of the stairs where I was. I woke them all and told them to get out of the house as fast as they could! The house was on fire!

It only took us about thirty seconds to get out of the house. All eleven of us (my mother-in-law was with us at the time) and our two dogs fled to our nearby fifteen-passenger van as I was calling 911. They were asking me questions like, "Is anybody still in the house, and how bad is the fire?" I had no idea. All I knew is that my brave husband was attempting to put out the flames with a fire extinguisher while I was trying to calm my baby, my kids, and myself.

And then, as the sirens were blazing through the neighborhood and the squad cars and trucks were pulling up, I realized that I was half-dressed. I had no pants on, and I was about to see the chief of police and fire department in my lace nightgown and underwear. Thankfully, it was right then that I saw my husband running out of the house with clothes for our son and me so I wouldn't have to face total humiliation. (I was on several city boards at the time, and the last thing I wanted was to have to work side by side next to a city official after he saw me in my not-so-flattering underwear).

The fire was contained quickly, but we were told that we could not go back into our house. While the damage was extensive, it could have been much worse. We packed a bag for all of us and drove to a local hotel, where eleven of us and two dogs tried to get some sleep.

The following day, we surveyed the aftermath. We called the insurance company, and I cried. I had no idea what was going to be our next step. We were not permitted to go back home until a professional cleaning crew came in and cleaned our entire house. We found out that meant so much more than just a few rags and some soap.

They had to remove every single item from our house. We had to gut Eli's bedroom because he was a baby, and we were told that anything he put into his mouth could not be *guaranteed* to be fully cleaned. Meanwhile, we needed a place to live for a month while all of this happened. The closest house that we found was well over an hour away.

That meant every morning, we would have to drive over an hour into town to take the kids to school, and then I would either return back to the rental house or camp out at the public library until school was over. This living arrangement was stressful, to say the least, and Eli was not a huge fan. The only saving grace was that the rental house had a giant jacuzzi tub. I spent several nights crying in the bath with a glass of wine. Our quasi-vacation home was also on a lake, so my husband and kids could take out a boat and go fishing. We were finding joy in unexpected circumstances.

Finally, we were given the *All Clear* to move back home. Sleeping in our own beds without an extra four hours of daily driving seemed like a dream. But then the real work began. Box after box after box of all of our stuff was being delivered to us. Hundreds of boxes were left in our garage for us to go through. It was like moving, except we didn't get any of the joys of picking out a new house, and our current house was now under renovation. The task was daunting, but we were able to press on.

It took us over a year to get back to normal and to get the things put away. But we did it!

During that time, my husband I had decided to become entrepreneurs. We researched ideas and viable businesses, and we made plan after plan to become business owners. And then, one day, out of the blue, it happened. We had a dream of an idea.

My husband loved working on jeeps and trucks, and he really wanted to own a shop where he could custom build auto parts for trucks. What can I say? I like big trucks, and I cannot lie. So, there we were, just over a year into our automotive business, struggling to live out our hopes of the American Dream, when then the unthinkable happened.

We were out to lunch celebrating a mostly successful summer with all of our crew. These four employees had become like family to us. I left my husband in the parking lot of the restaurant, kissed him goodbye so that I could go on with the rest of my afternoon. He called me less than five minutes later. He said, "the shop is on fire. You need to get over here!"

I told him that he had to be joking. But he wasn't. I raced across town to find the same ominous sight I had witnessed a few years back. Fire trucks, squad cars, and the street was blocked off. I watched as the crew went in and out of our building fighting that fire until it had gone out.

Everything that we owned and everything that we worked for was inside of that building. I watched and waited. Out of nowhere, I found myself on the ground in hysterics having a panic attack. I could hardly breathe, knowing that our dreams were going up into flames.

Eventually, the firemen gave us the *All Clear*, and we were able to enter the building. Everything had a thick layer of soot on it. However, it wasn't just all of our stuff. We had several customers that had their prized possessions in our building— expensive projects that we had been working on—all gone.

I couldn't even begin to fathom what the damage was. I just knew that it was going to be devastating. Now we knew what to do with this fire, having been experienced with the first. We made the calls and then just surveyed the damage.

I'd love to tell you, my dear readers, that this was an easy fix, and the insurance company came in and wrote a check, and all was well; unfortunately, that was not the case. It was hard, it was messy, and it was devastating.

The business was deemed a total loss. Everything was gone—including my personal jeep that was in our shop being used to take measurements for a project my husband was working on. There was nothing left to save.

My husband and I cried together. We just needed to sit and cry, you know? The next day, we got busy taking steps to rebuild. We spent months cleaning and clearing out all of the junk. That is when we made the decision. The show would have to go on! We would start again.

## Ringside Chat

At that time, I was reminded of the words of an old friend who told me that "you are always where you are meant to be. Even if you are in the middle of your house burning down, you are right where you are at. So, get out your roasting sticks and marshmallows and enjoy the moment."

That was the lesson that I learned through two fires, my dear ones. Remember, no matter where you are in life and no matter the circumstance, you are right where you are meant to be. You may not like what is happening right now in your life, but that doesn't mean that you cannot change everything.

After my house fire, my husband and I needed to remodel. I was able to pick out the exact flooring I had always wanted in my living room. We found beautiful stone to refinish my fireplace, and we were able to put in a brand-new insert so our fires could be cozier than before.

After our business fire, we changed locations, changed names, and even changed business plans to learn from the mistakes that we had made in the past and truly move forward from the fire.

After the great circus fire in Hartford, Connecticut in 1944, many people were too afraid ever to go back to a circus again. However, others went back and saw the value in the show continuing.

In 2004, a memorial was constructed at the same site of the circus fire, and it has been said that during the final Ringling Brothers tour in 2017 they returned to the very place where their worst nightmare had occurred.

You see, we all are faced with events that could devastate us and rock us to our very core—even completely ruin us with no way to go on from it. I have found that those who truly are able to embrace the *here and now*, and live in the moment will move on happier and healthier.

At the end of the day, it's not about how much you lose or how much you have, my dear friends; it is about how you live your life. Today, I challenge you to take a look around at your life and enjoy the very moment you are in—no matter the chaos, no matter the destruction, no matter how big the fire is blazing—just take it one moment at a time. This moment you are in, delight in it, and go roast some marshmallows.

You are loved.

# ··· CHAPTER 10 ···
# The Show Must Go On

NO ONE EVER expects tragedy to strike. It's not like you wake up one morning thinking *this will be the day that something terrible happens*. No, you wake up feeling that it will be *just another day*. You wake up, take a shower, get your coffee, and think that it will be the same old thing you have done day after day after day.

When I look back through circus history, I believe that these are the very same thoughts for many performers. How many times have they done the same daring act, day after day, performance after performance, without ever having a single issue? The performance: the same high wire act—with bicycles, the same stunt—performing the human pyramid, and the same juggling act—with fire and chainsaws.

The performers don't wait in anticipation for something terrible to happen, and neither do we. We just live our lives. But then, out of nowhere, the worst thing happens. Maybe someone was in the wrong place at the wrong time. Perhaps someone has a traffic accident, is in a burning building, or has an unexpected health challenge. Every day the news is filled with tragedies that have struck on just a typical day without warning.

• • •

The Flying Wallendas (the Great Wallendas) were known for their high wire acts—especially without a net. They hold the Guinness book of world records for high wire crossings over places like the Grand Canyon and Niagara Falls. However, the trick that made them famous was their human pyramid— the seven-person chair pyramid, to be exact.

The troupe of daredevil aerialists got up on that Tuesday, January 30, 1962, morning like any other day. I am sure they had their breakfast, stretched, and got their beautiful costumes on. Maybe they were laughing, making plans for after the show to head to downtown Detroit and enjoy the night. It's hard to say what happened that day.

The evening started without a hitch, and then up they went—four acrobats on the wire, holding their long stabilizing beams. Two more acrobats climb on top of them, and then finally, the last acrobat carefully climbs above them all and adds a chair for an extra thrill. They all work together like a well-oiled machine, having practiced this same trick many times before.

And then, it happened. Someone faltered ever so slightly, and it was all over. Three men fell to their death, and the others suffer severe injuries. A trick that had been done time and time again was now marred with tragedy.[1]

I can't imagine what it must have been like for their families and those audience members that day—to watch something so horrific.

And yet, how many times have we faced our own tragedies. I, too, have had my fair share of freak accidents, and close calls, and even a couple of fires. But it was a Monday in September that genuinely topped them all.

● ● ●

On September 23rd, 2019, I woke up like it was any other day. I posted on my Facebook to remind my friends that it was not Monday's fault if you have a bad day. We all make our own choices, and it is truly up to us how we deal with those choices.

I spent the day in a struggle. And like most typical Mondays, things were not going well. I don't blame *Monday*; it is just another day of the week, after all. Monday has no control over my attitude. However, everything felt a little off. Despite that, I was bound and determined to have a good day.

Morning dripping into lunchtime and lunchtime inched toward the afternoon. I can remember feeling that the bulk of the day had passed, and I just had to get through the afternoon. Suddenly, at 4:00 pm my husband called me. There was panic in his voice—it was not his typical sound.

He told me that I need to get to our shop as fast as possible—that it was crucial for me to return immediately. I had only left there minutes ago. I couldn't figure why this was such a big deal and why I needed to get back. I was still in the parking lot, honestly, and hadn't even made the turn from the driveway. So, I backed my car up and drove to where my husband was standing.

As I pulled up and saw my husband running at my car, I rolled down the window to my van. "Seriously, what?" I said to him, in kind of a snappy attitude.

"I don't know how to tell you this."

"Just tell me!" I huffed as my brain was racing on a thousand different things I had to do.

"Tell me!"

"Your brother... He's dead... Your dad just called me. You need to go home right now and meet a detective at the house."

How, in one moment, does a person deal with their entire life being flipped upside down?

I am not sure how I drove for the ten or so minutes it took to get to my house. I live about two miles from our shop, and on the way home, all I could do was try to wrap my head around the fact that my brother was no longer alive. That can't be done in just two miles. I sent my friend a voice text that was primarily hysterical and inaudible. I didn't even know what else to do.

I got home and sat and waited on my front steps. I sent my kids a text and told them that no matter what they saw out the front window to just stay inside of our house. I had no idea what I was about to endure in those following moments.

Within a few minutes of me arriving home, my husband pulled into the driveway. He told me that he didn't know any information. We sat there, just waiting.

An unmarked black SUV pulled up to my house, and a man got out. He was dressed casually, but his pants were muddy, and he looked worn out. His first words out of his mouth were, "I am sorry for your loss, I am sorry about your brother." As I sat there, realizing that this must no longer be a joke and trying to wrap my head around what was going on, I asked him what happened.

> "Your brother was murdered. Two shots to the back of the head."

"Your brother was murdered. Two shots to the back of the head."

In my entire life, I don't think I will forget those words; not only that but the shock that goes with it. My whole world changed in one instant, in the most unexpected and unpredictable way possible.

The questions started pounding against my head—the why's, the what-if's, the how's, the regrets, the anger, the grief—it all began. And then, at the same time that I was grieving, I had to call my siblings and let them know. I was the one that had to say to my sisters that my brother had been shot. There is no easy way to form those words.

For me, I just said them. Like ripping off a heavy adhesive band-aide again and again.

As the initial shock wore off, millions of emotions came flooding in like black darkness I tried to wrestle with—but how do you wrestle smoke? In the beginning, it was just sadness, emptiness, hallow. We did not have the name of the person who killed my brother, so it was constant heartache.

I'm the only sibling who lives near my parents, so I stayed busy helping make arrangements for my brother's memorial service. Now mingled in the entanglement of sadness was a feeling of uncertainty—of not knowing or ever knowing all the questions we were bombarded with from our minds. Grief would come in waves as we would find out details of what happened to my brother that night. My brain and heart would then flip again to the million questions that had no answers. In our wrestle of the dense black fog of sadness and grief, we became entangled in the gray uncertainty of unanswered questions—it is a feeling of suffocation and entrapment.

● ● ●

In life, tragedies are left with hundreds of unanswered questions, and ours was no different. The more details we were given, the more we would try to put together and gain some understanding about the who, the what, and the why of the incident.

After we were told of his murder, my entire family was feeling worn to the bone. How can you wake up each day and take care of life when so tragically, life had been so suddenly severed? I remember thinking, *how can everyone else rise up and go about their days when our world has halted in a smoldering crash?*

I wanted to shout at God to *stop the sun from rising and stop the world from spinning—a life had been lost—my brother!*

I felt more anger rise inside me!

*Did He (God) get it?*

*Didn't He understand?*

*Make the world stop!*

*Others need to see and feel our grief.*

*Others need to understand this wrestle of uncertainty.*

*Life SHOULD NOT go on!* But it did. *The show must go on.*

Five days later, Saturday, we held the memorial for my brother. We were not able to bury him at that time because we were told that "he [his body] was the best evidence for his case." We all sat around staring at a candle, a sickly yellow pool of light, his picture, a flag because he was a veteran, and some flowers were all we had to memorialize him with.

When you lose someone, you go through these questions, such as, *is this really real? How can this even be happening to us? Will we ever feel normal again?* That is where many of us sat that day. We had not seen his body. We were only given the fact that it was him based on his fingerprints. I wondered how many times my mom kissed those fingers, leaving their baby prints to linger on her lips?

The information was overwhelming.

My sister flew into town the day before the memorial and had to leave the day after. We spent every moment that we could together before we had to say good-bye. Everything felt fractured in our hearts. We would never all be together, in this life, again.

For two weeks, we sat waiting, wondering if there was to be a suspect. And then, with a crack in the case, the detective called us and told us that they had good news. I don't know how any information at this point could be considered good, but it was news of a suspect in custody.

We sat around my parent's living room with my sister on facetime as the detective told us the news. They had caught the killer. A woman. A woman? A woman from my brother's past had pulled the trigger twice, ending my brother's life. It was like I could hear the concussion of the double gunshots as he said it. Then I could see the smoke rising up towards her, but as the white smoke reached her face, it was smudged from my vision. I could not see the face of the killer no matter how many times that moment replayed in my head.

## Ringside Chat

And, unfortunately, this is where we sit today, as I write this. I would love to give you all the details, my dear readers, unfortunately, I cannot. Here is the thing, this chapter is not about the woman that killed my brother. It is about the tragedy that looms before us.

You see, there is more than just grief that is to be experienced during something so horrific as this. There is a chasm that opens up in our hearts. One where we live in a spiral of sadness and grief feeling like the world doesn't care, or has left us behind because they are on the other side of it—living. Living as if nothing has happened. And they are right! Nothing has happened—to them. The sun comes up, and life goes on—*the show must go on.*

So, how do you do that? How do you take all of the heartache, grief, and sadness and make it into something positive? How can death become positive? It can't, and yet it can. It's not about the event; it is about celebrating life—his life—his memories. Because the sun comes up each morning. I still have eight children who love me and depend on me to get myself out of bed and function because *the show* is going on for them.

Am I going to be there for them? *Yes,* I feel myself whisper. Because that is what this about right? Making your life the best life ever.

The first thing starts with one day at a time. It is a minute by minute, hour by hour, day-to-day scenario. I am not going to tell you overcoming any sort of tragedy is going to be easy. Sometimes you just have to take it moment by moment. Breath by breath.

Secondly, it is essential to feel all of the feelings as they bubble up, trigger, and consume hours of your life. This one is hard for a lot of people because oftentimes we don't want to feel the hurt, pain, heartache, and anger. We are ready to capture and stuff them away. We just want to ignore the feelings and say *we are fine.* Usually when someone says those words "I'm fine," they are, in fact, not fine.

I will tell you that it is much easier to feel what you are experiencing at the moment, then to stuff it down and ignore it. I know that it will not be comfortable for a while—grief never is, comfortable. So, we have to think of whatever emotion is presented to us; we will just walk, crawl, and sometimes run through it. Have yourself a good cry, take a hot shower, do whatever it is that helps you do to take care of yourself.

The more you allow yourself to feel what is being presented to you, the more it is actually purging the pain from you. I know—you are so excited, right? I wish there were a better answer, but there's not. Oh, sure, some think they can overcome it through pills, drinking, excessive eating, living, shopping, or even cleaning, but at the end of that activity, your pain is still there waiting for you; and now you are too tired to walk through it. How is that helping? Yeah, it's not. But here is the comfort. Millions of us have been through it. We are here beside you. I'm here. I get it. That is what this whole book is for—it's for you to know that I get it; I'm with you. I'm beside you.

Finally—the biggest thing of all—Forgiveness. Forgiveness is the one that takes the most work, but it has the most considerable pay-off—forgiveness for others and forgiveness of yourself.

Forgive yourself for the words you left unsaid. Forgive yourself for all of the times that you have beat yourself up over the thing that you are stressed out about—just forgive yourself. This is not an easy task, but it might be the most healing part of this journey. Tell yourself, I'm sorry, and I forgive you. Let yourself *let go*. How?

How? If you are living with a thousand regrets as I was, it's not easy to say the words, *I forgive me*. However, I am worthy to say it for myself. I am worthy of feeling love again. Yes, I know I can't talk to my brother face to face anymore. But I can revisit any hurt or wrong and say, *I forgive me*, and let it go.

The *blame game* is a real monster, and he will battle you to the death, to not have you say that. Sometimes he will even recruit other voices that start to swirl in your head, around and around, about what we *should-a, would-a, could*-a done. I *should have* had a better relationship with my brother. I *should have* told him I was sorry when I had the chance—when he was alive. I *should have* been the first to forgive for that petty argument, and not let it get in the way of our friendship together. Guilt, shame, blame—repeat! I didn't do any of that forgiving, and now he is dead. So, I revisit those painful moments. I sit in the uncomfortableness of the emotions and say *I'm sorry, and I forgive myself.*

I had to learn how to live in the space of forgiveness. I was crying bucket loads of tears every time I thought of my brother. There was guilt and shame for me not taking back all the crap I said about him when he was younger. A giant wall blocked my emotions from actually feeling the hurt and grief

I was experiencing. Forgiveness took months for me to work through because I believed I was the worst sister for never saying *I was sorry* to him and leaving things unsaid. What I discovered was, he did not have to be alive for me to apologize to him. I could say it each time the thought popped up. I had to make forgiveness a habit, and things started to improve.

After I forgave myself, I forgave him. I forgave him for the things that he said to me and all of the heartache that he caused me. I forgave him for being such an idiot sometimes and doing things that hurt my family. I simply forgave him for not being a better brother. Because who am I to judge it? Did I really know his circumstances? Honestly no. I will never feel the way that he felt.

● ● ●

As siblings, we did things together as a family, but his perspective is always different from mine. So, I really don't know how he felt about things. All I know is that I have to give him the benefit of the doubt —that he was doing the best he could for how he understood life to be. Maybe he thought he was a great brother. See expectations… they can get us because of our different perspectives.

When you get done forgiving yourself, then you have to forgive the one that hurt you.

I know, that is the hardest of all. Here I sit, telling you to forgive others, when I face this as my own daily hurdle. I will not even begin to tell you how much agony it causes me to know that I need to forgive the woman that has taken my brother's life. The act was selfish and senseless.

But the thing is, forgiveness is not for her; it's for me. The weight and the burden I would have to bear in order to carry eternal hatred would be far worse than if I let it go. I am *not asking* you to *go to the person* who hurt you, who played a part in your epic tragedy and tell them outright you forgive them.

What I am offering is that you just say it out loud—in the air, in your car, on a mountain, in the shower, or even, to God,

Maybe you are not even in that space yet. Perhaps you are only in the space where you can say it internally—and even that might be a stretch. It kills me that the woman who shot my brother sits one town away from me, free on bail, waiting for trial of the murder of my baby brother. But you know what else kills me? She is a mother, a daughter, a sister, and an aunt to someone—see perspective. Many lives were affected by the choice she made, and there is a LOT of people that need to experience forgiveness in this situation on both sides.

When you take the facts of the tragedy away and just put humanity's facts into play, forgiveness is easier. When faced with this kind of pain, there are layers upon layers, questions without answers, and pain without resolution.

Like most of us, the struggle is in the questions. And I will tell you, my friends, that the answers are in forgiveness. Whatever your challenge is today, whatever you are going through, know that there are others like you. Other people are facing similar struggles. You are not alone.

I think this, of the Flying Wallendas, too. How many *what-ifs* did they experience in the days that followed the great fall? What if I would have just had a steadier hand, what if we would have just used a net, what if… Those questions will always remain and never have an answer. So stop the madness—that's a three-ring circus you don't want to enter—stop asking that. Accept, forgive, and remember *the show must go on.*

I love you, my dear reader, and I believe in you.

# ··· CHAPTER 11 ···
# All Guts and Some Glory

WHEN I THINK about the circus, I think of some of the most epic people around. The stunts, the daring feats, the precision in timing, and the talent that has to be formed over the years is mind-boggling. Many of the performers who are in the circus have been there for generations. Year after year, these families are growing their trade, and they are teaching their new generation all about the circus.

Some of the acts that I consider to be most epic are the ones that involve great strength and height. Think about the performers who climb high into the air to walk across a tiny rope performing tricks, and the performers who fly with rhythmic precision, somersaulting, twisting and flipping over each other for the wide-mouth audience below.

Trapeze artist, rope and hoop flyers, and tight-rope walkers are the very essence of epic.[1] The definition of epic is particularly impressive or remarkable, grand in scale or character.[2] The tight-rope walkers simply walking from one side to another makes my heart jump—that alone is a fantastic feat. However, they don't stop there. They add chairs or jump ropes; they ride bicycles on the rope, and they carry one another on their shoulders. The acrobats prepare these stunts that leave us on the edge of our seats and gasping for breath as we watch.

And then for the grand finale, the truly most remarkable stunt of all, four or five people will make some human pyramid, all while being 50 to 100 feet up in the air. My mind is blown. My heart is in my throat until they make it back to their platforms safely. Their performance is a true definition of epic.

While I have never crossed a tight rope, or even so much as balanced a chair on my chin, I, too, feel as though I have done some epic things.

When I was thirty-five years old, I was diagnosed with Multiple Sclerosis. Those of you who don't know what that is, I'll break it down for you. MS is a chronic autoimmune disease that affects the brain and spinal cord, leaving lesions on these areas, thus causing symptoms like numbness, impairment of speech, fatigue, and blurred vision.[3]

> When I was thirty-five years old, I was diagnosed with Multiple Sclerosis.

I had just given birth to my son Eli, and I was spending a lot of time in the gym. Like most women, I felt pudgy from birthing a child and wanted a hot mom bod again. I belonged to a ladies-only gym, and we were in the midst of a program to shed twenty pounds in six weeks. Well, naturally, I wanted to get rid of that extra baby fat from the last sixteen years of carrying children, so I was *all in*.

I was going to the gym five days a week. I was kickboxing; I was lifting weights; I was doing cardio. I even learned how to hula hoop at thirty-five years old. And then when one day, when I was in the middle of a lifting set, my fingers felt numb. It felt like my hand *must have fallen asleep*, kind of discomfort. I didn't tell my trainer because I thought I must have pulled something, so I pressed on.

I had been a personal trainer for a few years, myself, so I knew about proper form, technique, rest, and all of those things that you should do to keep yourself healthy. I also had a goal in mind about what I wanted, so I just kept showing up to the gym. I wasn't going to let a few numb fingers and toes stop me from reaching my goals.

By the end of the next week, my legs, up to my waist, and both of my arms were experiencing extreme numbness. It was more than just the sleepy feeling; it was a constant throb and ache. I called my doctor, and they ran a lot of tests. There was a big concern as to whether or not I had a stroke at thirty-five years old after my son's birth. That is a common thing for women who have *geriatric pregnancies*.

One of the physical tests they repeated was where they would poke me with a pin going up and down my legs, all why while asking me questions and waiting for me to respond.

"Can you feel this?"

"Can you feel this?"

"How about here?"

Up and down, they poked me with a pin several times for several appointments. It was an extraordinary feeling, seeing someone dive a sharp pin in my leg and not be able to feel the poke.

Following the testing, the doctor told me that there wasn't anything to worry about. . . unless the numbness moved up past my waist. I stared at him for a good minute—like, really? He stared right back and replied to my *really* face by telling me if that numbness moved up past my waist, I should go straight to the emergency room. My head was racing with questions. *Why? Numbness all in my arms and lower body is ok, but if it happens above my waist, suddenly, it is an emergency?* This did not make sense, and I didn't feel reassured. I was an apprehensive mess.

I couldn't drive because I couldn't use my legs. My six-month-old baby needed to be carried around, and I couldn't feel my arms to do that. AGH! I was not the *sit around and wait for* kind of girl. I would hear him cry and get up and get him; it had to be done whether I could feel it or not. My husband was working nights at the time, so it wasn't like I could just lay and wait for someone to bring the baby to me. The struggle was real.

Within a week, I was in the emergency room as the numbness and tingling had spread. That's when I was scheduled to have an MRI done—phobia time! Two hours on my back in a tiny little machine, with all of the whirring, dinging, clicking, and popping going off, was torture. If you have ever had an MRI, you know exactly what I mean when I say it takes claustrophobia to a whole new level. If you have never had one, well, let's just say that I don't recommend them.

In the beginning, my insurance would only pay for one initial MRI, so when my test results came back, I was recommended to see a specialist. We drove an hour to the University hospital where the doctor we were seeing specialized in neurology and, more specifically, the disease Multiple Sclerosis.

I didn't need a doctor to tell me what it was. I already knew. I have an aunt and an uncle (who has now passed on) that have the disease. I saw my aunt go through many stages of it: annoying numbness, good days, bad weeks, and now she has to sit in either a wheelchair or push a rolling walker. Her brother, my uncle, by the end of his life, had an unrecognizable speech due to MS. He wheeled himself around in a motorized power chair, and eventually, he lost a leg due to complications between diabetes and MS. I knew what I was facing.

It had been over forty days since I had any normal feeling in my arms and legs. I wasn't even sure if I would ever regain feeling again. I knew another woman that always had that sense of tingling. And I wasn't sure what would happen or even what they would say. At that point, I wasn't sure if there were even going to be any answers.

The doctor that day informed me that I had some lesions on my spinal cord. To confirm the MS diagnosis, I would have to have another MRI, this time with the dye added to see if there were any enhanced lesions on my brain or spinal cord. Who is ready to throw me a claustrophobic party with that news? Right—no one!

It gets better. That MRI took close to three and a half hours. Three and a half hours of me not moving, laying still, on my back, which was causing me excruciating pain. They had given me some valium before I went into the machine, and I am not sure that it helped. What I do know is that it was the most extended three hours of my life, and I just kept saying to myself, you can make it another five minutes, and then I would count to 100—over and over and over. When that stopped working, I started thinking, dreaming, and doing everything I could except worry about the outcome because I knew that would not help me.

I got a call from the nurse about a week after the MRI. She wanted to tell me the results of my MRI but didn't want me to worry. *Well, babe,* I thought, *give it to me straight.* "It's Multiple Sclerosis."

For me, it was not a shocker. I had already guessed that. What I wanted to know was what was going to happen next? I was told there were many different treatment options and they all involved medication that would impact my ability to continue nursing Eli. I would need to stop doing that.

I know it sounds like, a duh thing: give up breastfeeding so that I can have treatments for MS. A few of you might judge me right now reading this, so let me share my perspective with you. Ladies, I had never had the opportunity to breastfeed before. I knew that he was my last child, and I wanted every moment I could spend with him, including breastfeeding. I mean, we only get one life. I told them that treatment would have to wait. They countered back with "the lesions would continue to grow and that my symptoms would worsen if I didn't start right away."

Sometimes, life just sucks. I knew what they said was true. I had read all of the packets of information they had given me. However, I knew that the medication was not a cure, so I was willing to take my time with Eli.

Miracles—I eventually regained feeling in my body. It was a daily struggle going through the flare-ups, however. There was a point when even walking from the couch to the bathroom was exhausting to me. One time I remember getting up off the couch, and the next thing I knew, I was on the floor with a twisted ankle because my legs had gone numb without me realizing it.

I spent almost two years that way, not working, just doing the *mom thing* while I chose Eli over my health. My doctor requested another MRI—really, again? Yes, three more hours in the tank of claustrophobia. I'd like to say that I was used to the machine and that it went better than my two other times, but I'd be lying to you. Nope, it was just as bad. After surviving the MRI, Eli and my husband brought me flowers—that was a bit of joy in the midst of all of the chaos. A few days later, the doctor called and told me to make an appointment to discuss the results of the testing.

He came straight out with it. My lesions were worse. I had more—more on my brain, more on my spine, and I needed to consider treatment. It had been two years since this *circus act* started performing in my life, and I had to step into the role of being the Ringmaster of my life—my health was on the line. I had to tell *the act* that Eli was no longer the reason I had put off my health. The Ringmaster won out. The

Ringmaster *cut the act,* and I started on a drug that involved me giving myself a daily injection.

Every single day I needed to put a needle up to my body, poke myself, and put these drugs into me. At first, I didn't think I could do it. In fact, I made my husband do it for the first two months. And then, one day, I just sucked it up and did it. I spent several months covered in welts until I could figure out the right thickness to shoot my subcutaneous fat. It wasn't easy. But eventually, I figured it out. Finally, the numbness stopped altogether. I had spent a good two years wallowing in this disease, and now, it was time for me to do something epic.

It was time for me to get my life back. What did I do—how did I start? I went for a walk. I made it three blocks. I looped around my neighborhood. Woot! Woot! The three blocks that I walked took me *seventeen minutes.* It was not what I would call epic by any means, but it was epic for me.

Immediately that negative voice popped up in my head. Wow! Seventeen minutes to walk three blocks—whoop! (Can you hear the sarcasm?) I mean, it is crazy. The very day I finally get up off the couch and take a walk, what happens? My head unleashes the negativity to start knocking down all of my efforts. I was frustrated because two years earlier, I had been bicycling every day, walking, and in the best shape of my life. And now, I could barely walk around the block. To add insult to injury, my husband and I had even been *cane* shopping!

However, I fought that negative voice. I started thinking about everything. Walking around the block was the most significant, grandest thing I could do in my life *at that moment.* (that was the key phrase—*at that moment*). So, I walked some more, and I walked for a few weeks, and then it turned into a few months.

With half a year of walking tucked under my belt, I decided to sign up for a challenge. I had been in a *runners' group* online that I had been following for several years before I ever got my diagnosis. On October 1st of that year, many in the *runner's group* were doing a fifty 5k challenge. That meant that every single day they were going to run a 5k for fifty days in a row. The farthest I had walked at that time was maybe two miles—a 5k is 3.1 miles.

I knew it was a little crazy, but I signed up. I put my mind to it and just said, *I am doing this.* Now, I knew that I was not going to be able to run. I could barely make my legs regularly work in any consistency. But I was going to do this challenge—I had to do it.

The first day, I set out with Eli in his stroller. He doubled as my walking buddy and a walking stabilizer. Pushing a stroller meant I could continue to ignore the need for a cane. I walked and walked and walked. Who knew that a 5k was *so* far? Seriously though, it felt like a marathon. It took me an hour and fifteen minutes to get done. I was not about to break any records with my 5k time, but I got it done.

Each day, I got up with the mindset that I was just going to do it. No matter how I was *feeling*, I was going to get after this goal. It wasn't easy. There were days that it rained, the wind blew, and I felt like quitting. But each day, I got up, I put on my workout clothes, and I just went for it.

Near the end of my challenge, there was a local race in my town. It was a 10k run for charity. That was double what I had been doing. As you can probably guess, I felt this was an incredible idea, so I prepared by *running* the course twice before race day. I believed that I could totally do it in the race because I had already done it. One of my friends signed up with me, and we chose to get after it.

Just to clarify, when I say *I ran the course*, It was more like *I wogged* the race course. *Wogging* is the cross between a jogger and a walker, but it was still something. I knew I would never break records, but that was not my goal. My goal was to be a part of the race.

Race day came, and my friend, Eli, and I all started on the course. It was pretty hard. My *wogging* mile after *wogging* mile, I placed my feet in front of each other. This was totally mindset time for me (who would win—negative or positive), and I dug in deep. When we came up the final hill to cross the finish line, I was so excited. It was the finish. It was there—right there! I had done something HUGE. I not only completed my fifty 5ks in fifty days, but I also did a 10k. I came in *dead last*! BUT I did it.

At that moment, this was epic! My performance was in the spotlight of my life. It was my circus performance. My crowd was cheering, the other acts were cheering, and although I might not be some great circus performer or some movie star, at that moment, I had cross that *tight-rope*. I was on the other side of the platform, and like a queen, I took my bow and relished in the applause of the entire circus.

I didn't stop there! I wanted more! I wanted to truly see how far I could go to beat this disease. When you have an autoimmune disease without a cure, there are only two things that you can do.

1. You can face your day with disappointment, or
2. You can get on with your life and live your best life.

That is what I wanted to choose for myself.

Not long after that, I found a race designed for all women of any shape, size, or ability to do a half marathon. I was intrigued. 13.1 miles is a long way. That's from my house to the next town over! It's especially far for someone who doesn't have control of her legs at any given time.

But I wanted to try. I wanted to prove to myself that I could do anything. Naturally, I did what any good woman would do; I wrote an impassioned letter to the race creator applying to be a race day ambassador. I told them of my struggles with MS and wanted to be chosen as the face for every woman to let them know that they can do anything.

I didn't think I would get chosen to be one of the ambassadors, but I was! An ambassador meant that I would have to *run* the race. Ok, I thought, *I can wog*, and that is where I will start. Slowly and painfully, I began training and practicing to *wog* thirteen miles. Yes, I was slow, and there were days I was sure I saw a few turtles pass me on my journey, but I did it.

The time came for me to show up on race day to prove to the world, and myself, that I could do something of this magnitude—a half marathon.

I got up that morning with great anticipation. I was running the checklist in my head, getting all stoked and excited, and then WHAM! The fear set in. Every *what-if* that I ever carried around was weighing me down. I had looked at the weather report and found out it was going to be incredibly hot. Ok, heat—what's a little heat? I had to make a choice, give in to the fear or go? (Just as a side note, I wasn't prepared for the heat the way I thought I was).

I thought to myself; *this is no big deal. If I can be the mother to eight children, I can do anything.* I felt my shoes underneath me, had my number pinned to me, hundreds of other runners were around me, and I looked straight ahead. The starting buzzer went off! I started on my journey through the streets of Madison, Wi. The first couple of miles were comfortable, and I kept on smiling.

*Wog, wog, wog,* I thought—*just keep wogging!* It was working—miles were going underneath me. My mindset was overcoming the negativity. Somewhere mid-way through the race, though, I began to lose feeling in my legs. *It's ok. It's ok,* I kept thinking. Step, step, step, step. My mind jumped to the thought. *You don't have Eli. Where's the stroller for your stabilizer?* I knew the answer. They were not here. Step, step, step, step. Just keep stepping. I just needed to press on.

At mile six or so, a woman caught up with me, and we began to walk/running through the streets together. That helped. She was like that breath of fresh air to help you keep going. But, by mile nine, I was ready to give up this circus act. I was done. I felt my feet respond to the negativity, and at one point, they stopped. I was hitting a wall, both physically and mentally.

Guess what happened? I told myself, *how stupid I was for even thinking that I could do something as unique as this*. Gulp! It's true—I started giving in to the negative voices --the shouts from the crowd—I even felt like they were *booing* me. Really, Angela—at a time like this, you are going negative? And then, like the clowns in the circus, several women stopped and talked to me. One offered to go the next mile with us, one offered me a power bar, one started making jokes and distracting me from the pain and misery I was in. These women rallied around me so I could keep going the next step. (See, clowns are a great thing).

At mile eleven, though, my body started telling me that it was time to be done. I was going slower and slower. By this time, I had lost all feeling in my legs and arms. I wasn't sure how I could even go on any longer. But step by step, I did go on, with all of the strength I could gather, I pictured myself inching towards the finish line just like the thousands of tight-rope walkers who can see the other side of the platform—just a few more steps!

One mile before the finish line, a couple of my friends (who were actual runners) came flying past me. They had a later start time than me. They were nearly lapping me. As they checked in on me, I knew that I was fading very quickly and that I would need medical attention by the time I crossed the finish line. They promised to run ahead and have someone ready.

With dedication and perseverance, I crossed the finish line. The woman who joined up with me at mile six had to hold my arm up in the air to high five the people standing cheering for me there. The medics met me on the other side of the line and carried me to the medic tent.

I tried to pretend that I was fine, and after 10 minutes or so, I got up and walked into the air-conditioned building nearby. I promptly collapsed in the hallways. I was not ok! I was overheated and dehydrated.

I earned myself a ride by ambulance to the nearest hospital. Someone called my husband to meet me, and the rest is a blur. I am told they packed me in ice and pumped me full of medications and fluids. I felt foolish that I needed my husband to rescue me on my epic journey to prove that I could beat this disease.

● ● ●

Just as the flying trapezes artist knows a safety net means you get to fly another day, my hubby was my safety net. He was there to pick me up. It made me remember that even the best tight rope walkers and trapezes artists fall sometimes. They pick themselves back up and do it again. They not only do it too, but they also go for bigger stunts, better stunts, and something even more epic than the one before.

After what I could only see as my epic failure of ending up in the hospital following a half marathon, a woman had reached out to me. She talked to me about what I had accomplished while having MS. She only saw accomplishment, all guts, and some glory. I was confused and humbled by her words. Dang! I didn't fail. I finished.

She continued to reinforce that I was a finisher, and then she shared with me that there was a run that was happening the following year—a cross country run. It was a relay to raise money and awareness for people with MS. Most of the runners were cross country runners that participated in events like Ironman or weekly marathons. And occasionally, they would have someone with MS sign up. She felt that I could be that person.

Suddenly my mind shifted from failure to winner! I wanted to do it. I wanted to be a part of this cross-country run. For the second time, I sent my passionate letter to the race coordinator. She received the letter and interviewed me. In the interview, I told her that "I was not a runner," "I can barely run a 15-minute mile." I also revealed that I collapsed the last time I did a half marathon. However, the following sentence I said was, "You should choose me because I want to prove that I *can* do this." That did it. I got the invitation in the mail a few weeks later.

Now, how to tell my husband? (I know, slight detail I needed to fix.) Well, he must love the circus show I have because although he thought I was crazy, he was super supportive. Together, we quickly worked out the logistics of how he would be *managing our circus* without me for twelve days, and then I got to work. I needed an accountability runner, and I met up with someone who could run circles around me, yet every day we met for our *run*.

I was slower than molasses in January on a cold Wisconsin winter day, but I was out there doing it. I was not getting any faster. However, I was staying consistent—slow and steady. My body also seemed to understand that this getting up and going for several miles a day was the new normal. I was no longer losing feeling in my legs and arms daily, which was a good sign.

The training and the conversations I had with my body went something like this.

"Yeah!"

"Ug!

"Wait…"

"Sure!"

"I think I can, I think I can, I think I can…"

"Kill me!"

"Just one more step, just one more step!"

Needless to say, it was brutal. There was a time that I considered quitting, but I didn't have it in me. I knew that this was something that I had to do. After speaking with the coordinator and planning the route that would best serve me and not kill me in the process, the plan was for me to run 100 miles across Colorado in seven days. The SAG team (support and gear) would be alongside me for snacks, water, first aid, change of clothes, and anything else I might need. (I don't want you to worry that I was doing this without support.) I absolutely had the best team, and they were patient with me.

The first morning we started early to beat the sun, and I honestly thought I was insane the entire time. I was hot, my body was exhausted from all of the training, but the roads were flat. However, I had still not prepared enough for this race. I don't know what I was thinking signing up for a cross-country run. I mean, there were days I could barely walk.

I was only able to go twelve miles the first day. I could see the disappointment in the SAG crew's eyes. I was not their typical marathon runner. I was nothing like the rest of the team at all. Usually, the rest of my teammates went out and ran their marathon in a few hours and then had the rest of the day off. It took me over three hours to finish twelve miles. I guess my SAG team was really earning their pay with me.

We stayed in a camper. After my twelve-mile day, I went back to the camper, where I showered and sulked. I knew that I would have to pick myself up out of this stinking way of thinking and put my mind to work. I told myself daily that I could do anything, and it was time to believe it.

The days were hot and incredibly long. The weather was in the mid-'90s, and there was very little shade on the road that I was running on. By midday, I was sunburned, had excruciating pain in my legs, and missing my family. I knew that giving up was not an option, but I wanted it to be after the day's run. I could have asked one of the SAG team members to take a few miles for me. But, as soon as I thought that, I just knew I couldn't ask for that. I was unwilling. I knew I had to keep going. I had to conquer the great unknown of this disease if I planned to win the battle.

On the morning of day five, I still had forty-six miles to go over the next three days. I was going to have to push through. The first step I took that day, I knew something was wrong. My knee was killing me. The first SAG stop was at mile four, and it took me way too long to get there. I took some ibuprofen and kept going.

My knee was swollen, and every step I took felt like razors slicing me through my legs. Tears were rolling down my face by the time I made it to the eight-mile mark. I didn't think that I could go any further, but the SAG team encouraged me to press on. I had too many miles that still needed to be covered, and it was getting hot out. It took me almost two hours to finish those last four miles to make it to twelve miles. I needed to stop.

There was no way I could keep going with the pain that I was experiencing. We drove back to the camper, and I showered and stretched out. The talk was that later that evening, I would go out and do four more miles to have fewer miles over the last two days. I decided that I would just wear my favorite sandals instead of running shoes. I would give my legs a break and a different pair of shoes.

My sandals felt great! My knee pain was gone wearing my sandals. I couldn't explain it, but I was feeling so much better. I even started running. Actual running! When I showed up at the SAG stop faster than they expected, my team was surprised when I told them that I wanted to keep going!

That day I ended up going twenty miles. The farthest I had ever gone in one day. All that was left was for me to accomplish one marathon. And I still had two days left.

The following day, I got up, and I set out in my tennis shoes. We brought my sandals along just in case, but I had wanted to at least start in my shoes that were designed for running. After the first four miles, I changed my shoes, and I decided that I would finish this thing TODAY. I wanted to have a marathon under my belt.

At that point in my life, the most challenging thing I had done was give Michael up for adoption, and this felt *even harder* than that moment. It was like I had to draw upon that strength to finish this. I just kept walking. I kept putting one foot in front of the other without stopping. I ignored the pain in my legs and just kept going.

We stopped for lunch and a small break, and then I told the team I would finish the relay that afternoon. They told me that I could only go until dark, and then for safety, they would have to pull me off the road. Everything in me wanted to be finished that day. I really wanted to get up early the next day and drive the fourteen hours home and surprise my husband.

The darkness was setting in, and I could see the SAG vehicle up ahead waiting for me. When I got there, they said, "you have one mile left. You can do it now or first thing in the morning." I knew without a shadow of a doubt I was going to finish the race right then.

I cried the entire last mile. I had *Fight Song* playing on my radio, and the words were playing through me with every step I took.

"...I don't care if nobody else believes,
cause I've still got a lot of fight left in me."[3]

I crossed the finish line and laid down on the ground, and sobbed like a baby. I did it! I had done a marathon with Multiple Sclerosis. I still had a feeling in my legs; I was not headed off to the hospital. I felt great. It was then that I realized how genuinely epic I was. That I was able to accomplish anything I set my mind to do.

It was like carrying five people on my back while crossing the tight rope without a net. I had done the impossible.

Except, it was possible. It gave me great strength and mindset that whatever I set out to do, I could do. No matter what.

## Ringside Chat

I came home from that epic journey, changed and with a renewed spirit. That was just a few years ago, but it seems like a lifetime.

I decided on that long drive home from Colorado to Wisconsin while I cried and laughed about what I had accomplished, that I was no longer going to carry the weight and the burden of being a patient of MS. Now I rarely claim that I have this disease any longer.

I found some alternative treatments that I take, and I very rarely have MS symptoms. I treat myself to living my best life and carrying on with the *CAN-DO* attitude. I continue to believe that I can create and accomplish epic things if I just put my mind to it.

So, I challenge you, my dear reader; whatever you face today, whatever your challenges are, believe you can do it. You can live your best life. Whatever that looks like for you. Sometimes that means getting rid of the safety net and going for the truly epic things. And sometimes epic simply means going for a walk that is just three blocks long.

Anyone that ever did anything tremendous and epic in their life didn't start out doing epic things. No, they started small and built up to it. Just like I have done and many others who have gone before me—so can you!

You can start now. You can start today. On this epic journey, we call life and go after your dreams. I believe in you.

# ··· CHAPTER 12 ···
# Your Place in The Circus

THE MOVIE, *THE Greatest Showman* came out at the end of 2017. It was hardly talked about, barely even advertised, and then, something incredible happened. The Hugh Jackman movie became a huge sensation.[1]

This movie is about the Great PT Barnum. While it is a mostly fictional movie, PT was a showman extraordinaire and truly loved oddities. One of the movie's main characters, Lettie Lutz, is the singing-bearded-fat lady—like our dear Dolly Dimples from the beginning of this book.

Lettie feels invisible and is deeply hurt by the people who laugh at her. She finds comfort in knowing that PT finds her beautiful, and she finds a home amongst the other misfits like her.

The movie takes a turn when PT is obsessed with making an *honest dollar* and hires a beautiful woman to partner with to run a show. The circus freaks are tossed to the side, and almost forgotten.

In this scene, Lettie Lutz has her break though moment. The song that would go on to be a best-selling song from this movie.[2]

She sings about how she is not a *stranger to the dark*, and that her oddity needed to be hidden because no one wanted to see her *broken parts*. The shame in her life builds up, and it breaks her heart. She convinces herself that she is not worth living. (Ladies! This is real pain here—tears fall even as I write this).

If you are now singing those lyrics in your head, you are my people! This song could be an anthem to my heart. How many times did I feel as though I was too scarred for the masses? How many times did I feel ashamed because my story was too much for people?

I remember speaking to an audience of foster parents. I told my story of the challenges that I had faced. I was open, I was brutally honest, and I held nothing back. A week later, I received feedback from the company explaining that my story was just too much for other foster parents to hear, and I would not be welcomed back because, "I was too honest."

I spent several hours feeling sad—even bruised by these words. I had wanted so desperately to make an impact for foster parents, and then there I was, being *too much again*. I felt like I was constantly in an imbalance from being *too much* for people or *not enough*.

And then, like a healing balm, the words from the movie played in my head again. She makes *a choice* not to allow them to break her. She has a place, she is loved, and belongs to them… and then my mind recalls the last phrase, "For we are glorious!"

## Ringside Chat

My dear ones, hear me when I say this to you. You are not too much for anyone. Whatever challenge you are going through right now. You are not too broken, because you CANNOT be broken.

You might be bruised, you might be scarred, but you are not broken.

I have a lot of different kinds of friends. Just like the circus has many different acts/performances. I surround myself with women of all types: I have friends who are walkers, runners, and yoga people (and not just I-have-yoga-pants people). I have friends that are stay-at-home moms, businesswomen/moms, homeschool moms, dog moms, and so forth.

Here is an example of my runner mom's friends. I have friends that don't just like to run—they run a lot! They are the kind of people that say, "Eh, I am just doing a marathon this weekend, no big deal." And I am jealous. I have friends who do Ironman's. I know one woman who has done *NINE*—Nine Ironman's!

I have friends who are moms—just moms. Well, there is never *JUST* a mom. It is hard to call a person who stays home every day managing their entire household with tiny tyrants for bosses as *JUST* anything. But they are stay-at-home-moms—and they rock it well.

I have friends who are homeschool moms, and every single day my head spins as they post about their five kids and what they did for their latest history lesson. Most of the time, they are learning about people I have never even heard of before and are building projects of places that only exist in my mind.

I have friends that own businesses, like myself, and often times I find myself comparing myself to them. I am wondering if they are better at business than me—more successful even. I compare myself to these other women because I often think, "man, you have it all together."

Usually, one of us ends up having a conversation with the other person about how something has gone wrong, and that is when I think, "well geez, all of us are just barely holding our shit together. Who knew?" I am just like those women!

I have friends who have been through extreme trauma. I have friends that the biggest trauma that they have ever had was what they should make for dinner and watch tonight on Netflix. It doesn't make either of these women, more or less.

You see, we have all been through something. You've all read how I was twenty-three years old, and I had already lived more life than most forty-year-old women. I want to share about some women I knew. Women I judged when I was younger.

You see, I knew these girls were the most perfect girls I had ever seen. They dressed ultra conservative in jean skirts and turtlenecks. They spoke softly. Every time we went anywhere together, they brought something homemade. In my mind, they were perfect. I had always dreamed of being like them.

I was fairly torn up as an individual at that time in my life. I had been married and divorced. I had three small kids that I was always toting around. I could barely afford to feed my family, let alone dress us decently. I was a single mom, and I was envious of so many people who I thought had a *perfect life*.

One day, I remember talking to them and saying that "they would never understand what my life was like." They replied, "You know what? We spit, we run, and we wear pants sometimes and don't think you are the only sinner." (Yes, that was an actual conversation I had with someone). In my mind, I thought if they only knew how much of a *sinner* I was, their hair would curl up like my bad 1980s perm I got in the fifth grade.

As we grew older, I discovered that some of these same women struggled to have children. They fought with their husbands just like I did. They were not taken seriously in their jobs. They struggled living life in the *real world* because they had been sheltered when they were younger. Their mom, who I had placed had on a pedestal for raising such amazing women, shared with me that she was in a loveless marriage. She only stayed because she thought it was the *right thing to do*. It was then that I learned how to find deep compassion for women—all women.

I learned that as women, even if our lives are so catastrophically different, we were all just women. We are all the SAME! We are just women trying to make it in the world. Women, trying to do and be our true selves and live in our purpose.

● ● ●

We need women to find other women and to love other women—for us to love each other. For me, I created something called *Pie Night* amongst my friends. *Pie Night* is a place where we can gather together as women and truly let our guards down. This is a safe space. It is not to degrade one another or even those we are struggling with. It is a place where you can share and talk things out. *Pie Night* is that place. It is a no judgement zone.

Here we can talk about all the topics we want (husbands, kids, church, work, pets, etc). What is said here *stays here*. It is a safe place to belong because sometimes we have a lot of emotional vomit spewing, and that is fine. We all are a part of it, and we all clean it up. Open and honest, without judgment of others. We bring all of our own oddities here. We are never too much for each other. We are just right the way we are, and who we are. This is that place.

By creating this space and place, I started to understand relationships at a deeper level. I was made aware of who I was and that I brought value to my community. I was valued here. And now, I can bring this to other women, so that they see who they are. Because they are glorious! Because WE ALL ARE GLORIOUS!

I have been delighting in the differences of these women ever since I created *Pie Night*. I delight in other women's journey because it is in and through the journeys of these women, I have learned so much. I have learned grace, strength, and I overcome hardships. I have become a better juggler, tight rope walker, and even a Ringmaster through the lives of others.

My dear friends, I have a question for you. When you look at the women you spend your time with, are you in judgment of them, or are you finding joy in their journey? I hope it is the latter because the journey is hard, my friends. Your journey is not my journey, and it never will be. It will always be your journey, but I can be beside you, listening to you, showing empathy, and loving you.

There is a saying to *not judge a person until you walk a mile in their shoes*, but I ask you, do you need to walk in anyone else's shoes? Can we agree that your shoes are your very own, and someone else's shoes are theirs? Your shoes fit you exactly like they should. They are not too big or too small. They are exactly as they should be.

My dear friends, I hope that you understand that you were created for a purpose. You were created for joy. You were created for greatness. You were created for love. You were created and designed perfectly and uniquely you. Apologize for nothing!

And the my final words from the dear Lettie.
"I'm not scared to be seen.
I make no apologies.
This is me."[3]

## ··· EPILOGUE ···

# Enjoy Your Show

IT'S SEPTEMBER, THE air is crisp, and the leaves have just started changing into magnificent colors of orange, gold, and a deep cranberry color. The summer of the circus is over and my children have all gone back to school.

My children have left for college, high school, and my tiny Ringmaster, Eli—the baby I always wanted and dreamed of, is now five years old. He just started kindergarten.

I drive to my beloved Circus World's grounds, where they are only open for limited fall hours. I sit on the bench and take in the music that plays over the loudspeakers. I have the freedom to walk through the exhibits, uninhibited by my children, and look at all of the posters and circus paraphernalia from days gone past.

The Big Top tent, usually can be seen from the road throughout the summer months, is now gone, and only the empty cement slab remains. My favorite girls, the elephants, have gone home to their sanctuary in Oklahoma to prepare for another traveling season away from Baraboo.

The performers have "moved on down the road," as they like to say in the circus. The season is over.

It's is a new season—the time to rest for the circus. And for you, a new season of your life. Your season of life will constantly be changing. It will always be flowing. Your circus will always look different as the years go on.

Things will change. Kids will grow up from babies to toddlers, to teens, and adults. They will grow and change and eventually leave and go on to have babies of their own. Even in the short span of five years, your life will look different than it does right now.

In five or ten years, everything could be different. The years change us. The seasons change us. It is our choice if we want to change with them, just like we did this summer: to jump a ride on a circus train and go with the flow, or to stay stagnant stuck in misery.

The circus reminds us of family and all of the changes that come with it—moving and growing with the generations. I guarantee the circuses of our grandparents are not the ones that we see today. Instead of the daylong event that came to town on a train, we find the entertainment in movies, television, video games, and occasionally a live performance that lasts 90 minutes. There are so many circus performers that are often five and six generations of the circus family. But whether they are old or new performers, they have to adapt to the change just like everyone else.

While this season of the circus is now over, and I sit on a dusty bench trying to imagine the Big Top from just a few weeks ago. I breathe in the cool air and the faint memories of my summer I spent with my children at the circus. I am reminded that the circus will be back in just a few months when the winter is over and that my children are growing into their own new seasons.

This life, this circus life, is everything that we will ever have. The joys, the tragedies, the silly, and the sad. And so, my dear friends, embrace your life. Enjoy all of the chaos, and all of the seasons of change.

And no matter where you are in life, as it is said at the end of every show,

*"MAY ALL YOUR DAYS BE CIRCUS DAYS!"*[1]

# End Notes

Introduction:
1. Wikipedia. 2021. "Circus World Museum." Last modified, 30, Jan 2021. https://en.wikipedia.org/wiki/Circus_World_Museum

Chapter One:
1. Wikipedia. 2020. "Celesta Geyer." Last modified, 16, July 2020. https://en.wikipedia.org/wiki/Celesta_Geyer

Chapter Two:
1. Wikipedia. 2021. "Freak Show." Last modified, 20, Jan 2021. https://en.wikipedia.org/wiki/Freak_show
2. Wikipedia. 2021. "Chang and Eng Bunker." Last modified, 1, Feb 2021. https://en.wikipedia.org/wiki/Chang_and_Eng_Bunker.

Chapter Three:
1.  Wikipedia. 2021. "Katie Sandwina." Last modified, 6, Feb 2021. https://en.wikipedia.org/wiki/ Katie_Sandwina

Chapter Five:
1.  Wikipedia. 2021. "Ringling Bros and Barnum." Last modified, 17, Jan 2021. https://en.wikipedia.org/wiki/ Ringling_Bros._and_Barnum_%26_Bailey_Circus
2.  Wikipedia. 2021. "Elephant." Last modified, 26, Jan 2021. https://en.wikipedia.org/wiki/Elephant

Chapter Six:
1.  Ben Bromley. "The Pursuit of Happy-ness: Clown Wins Gem Award." Baraboo New Republic. 25, June 2015. https://www.wiscnews.com/ baraboonewsrepublic/news/local/the-pursuit-of-happy-ness-clown-wins-gem-award/article_eb01af77-0f31-5be9-948d-9fd01816d605. html?fbclid=IwAR2ahOdlcJIZySiRtDfcmx3dm-CIg3_kNuXMj7cvfcng-zHdqi7qs-81uYvs
2.  Wikipedia.2021. "Ringling Brothers Circus." Last modified, 12, Jan 2021. https://en.wikipedia.org/wiki/ Ringling_Bros._and_Barnum_%26_Bailey_Circus

Chapter Seven:
1.  Wikipedia. 2021 "Ringmaster." 20, Jan. 2021 https:// en.wikipedia.org/wiki/Ringmaster_(circus)

Chapter Eight:
1.  Wikipedia. 2021. "Juggling." Last modified, 15, Feb 2021.https://en.wikipedia.org/wiki/Juggling

Chapter Nine:
1. Wikipedia. 2021. "Hartford Circus Fire." Last modified, 25, Jan 2021. https://en.wikipedia.org/wiki/Hartford_circus_fire

Chapter 10:
1. Wikipedia. 2020. "The Flying Wallendas." Last modified, 30, Oct 2021. https://en.wikipedia.org/wiki/The_Flying_Wallendas

Chapter 11:
1. Wikipedia. 2021. "Acts of the Circus." Last modified, 11, Feb 2021. https://en.wikipedia.org/wiki/Circus
2. Wikipedia. 2021. "Epic." Last modified, 16 Feb 2021. https://en.wikipedia.org/wiki/Epic
3. Rachel Platten, Dave Bassett. "Fight Song." Fight song. First edition. Single. Columbia Records. 2015

Chapter 12:
1. Condon, Bill. Bricks, Jenny. Michael Gracey. 2017. Musical/Drama. Disney
2. Keala Settle. Benj Pasek. Justin Paul. "This is Me." The Greatest Showman Movie 2017. Single. Atlanta Records. 30, Oct 2017.
3. Keala Settle. Benj Pasek. Justin Paul. "This is Me." The Greatest Showman Movie 2017. Single. Atlanta Records. 30, Oct 2017. https://www.lyrics.com/lyric/34576181/This+Is+Me

Epilogue
1. Ryan, Jack. "Obituary: May All Your Days Be Circus Days." Los Angeles Times, 2016. 26, Aug. https://www.legacy.com/obituaries/latimes/obituary.aspx?n=jack-ryan&pid=181227171

Dearest,

I hope you have enjoyed this circus adventure as you have joined me in the details of my life. I want you to know why I share all of these most intimate details with you. I genuinely want you to know that you are not alone in life. Life is so hard sometimes, and I get that. BUT DO NOT LOSE HOPE.

You are an amazing, valuable woman, and I believe in you.

If you find yourself struggling, please reach out. I am here for you. My email address is choosetoday366@gmail.com.

This is my personal email for you to send me a message when you feel like giving up. I will encourage you. I will be here for you. I will help you find some strength for you to endure your circus for another day.

You can also reach me through my website, www.choosetoday366.com

There I offer courses and coaching to help move you to a place of discovery and self-love. Your growth is important to me.

You matter to me.

I love you,
Angela Witczak

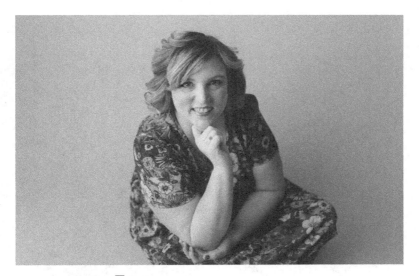

# I love you.

choosetoday366@gmail.com

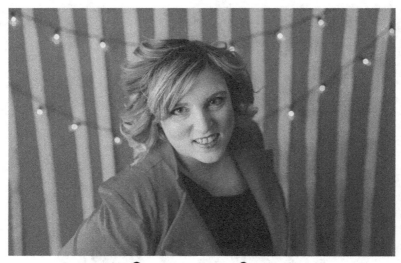

I believe in you

CPSIA information can be obtained
at www.ICGtesting.com
Printed in the USA
BVHW041058290421
606035BV00004B/38/J